The Jossey-Bass Health Series brings together the most current information and ideas in health care from the leaders in the field. Titles from the Jossey-Bass Health Series include these essential health care resources:

Profiting from Quality

Profiting from Quality

Outcomes Strategies for Medical Practice

Steven F. Isenberg and Richard E. Gliklich,

Editors

Jossey-Bass Publishers • San Francisco

Jossey-Bass books and products are available through most bookstores. To contact Jossey-Bass directly, call (888) 378–2537, fax to (800) 605–2665, or visit our website at www.josseybass.com.

Substantial discounts on bulk quantities of Jossey-Bass books are available to corporations, professional associations, and other organizations. For details and discount information, contact the special sales department at Jossey-Bass.

 Manufactured in the United States of America on Lyons Falls Turin Book. This paper is acid-free and 100 percent totally chlorine-free.

Library of Congress Cataloging-in-Publication Data

Profiting from quality : outcomes strategies for medical practice / [edited by]
    Steven F. Isenberg . . . [et al.].
       p.   cm.
    Includes bibliographical references and index.
    ISBN 0-7879-4624-9 (hc : alk. paper)
    1. Medicine—Practice—Quality control—Economic aspects. 2. Medical care—
Quality control—Economic aspects. 3. Quality assurance—Economic aspects.
4. Outcome assessment (Medical care)—Economic aspects. I. Isenberg, Steven F.
    [DNLM: 1. Quality Assurance, Health Care—economics. 2. Outcome Assessment
(Health Care)—economics. W 84. 1 P9639 1999]
RA410.5.P759—dc21
DNLM/DLC
for Library of Congress   99-12557
                                                                                                        CIP

FIRST EDITION
HB Printing   10 9 8 7 6 5 4 3 2 1

Contents

Preface

This book is intended for physician leaders, from physician executives in health care organizations to practitioners who are leading small practices. It is intended as a guidebook to the emerging sciences of health measurement, quality management, and information technology, which collectively form a new discipline called *outcomes* that may fundamentally change the practice of medicine. Yet in the decade since Paul Ellwood (1988) introduced the term *outcomes management* and the concept that continuous feedback loops of outcomes data would provide the means to improve the health care system over time, widespread adoption has been slow. Some of the reasons have been the need for further development in the field, an emphasis on cost rather than quality, and the need for information technology to make outcomes measurement less burdensome in actual practice. But another reason has been concern among physicians for how the data will be used and who will pay for their collection. The future of the outcomes movement relies on physician participation, and physician participation is contingent on appropriate incentives for their efforts. Profiting from quality can present itself in many forms: reduced costs, higher revenue, improved marketing, and better patient care. In this regard, participation can provide a competitive advantage.

The conclusion of the contributors to this book is that the desire for outcomes information from a multitude of stakeholders will push the field of outcomes forward. There exists a window of opportunity now for physicians to lead the charge. The reasons to participate in outcomes assessment that exist today need not be all altruistic. The argument is made throughout this book that patients, physicians, and organizations all can and should profit from quality, and case examples are provided. Other industries, both manufacturing and service, have invested heavily in measuring and improving quality and have reaped the rewards. The health care industry is unlikely to be different.

This book is divided into three parts. All of the chapters in Part One were written by Uwe E. Reinhardt and May Tsung-mei Cheng, who explore from an economist's perspective a number of contentious issues surrounding the quality of health care. Chapter One develops the concepts of the macroquality of the health care system, which includes the quality of life of providers as well as patients, and microquality, which refers to the results of medical treatments and processes. Chapter Two adds empirical evidence to suggest that no health system today is properly accountable for the quality of health care it delivers nor does any come close to maximizing the quality of health care for given levels of expenditures.

Part Two focuses on outcomes as a method to examine the microquality of health care and serves as a primer on the principles and practice of outcomes measurement and management. Chapter Three provides a basic overview of outcomes management. Chapter Four explains the necessary principles of clinical research design that must be applied for useful real-world measurement, and Chapter Five provides a working knowledge of the development and limitations of the tools themselves, the outcomes measures. Chapter Six addresses the value of measuring patient satisfaction, and Chapter Seven outlines the practical steps of every outcomes study and the pitfalls to be avoided. Chapter Eight explores the role of new technologies, including the Internet, in facilitating outcomes management, and Chapter Nine describes the role of data management in maximizing the value of outcomes and quality data.

Part Three focuses on how and why medical practices should implement outcomes measurement: that it is ultimately in their best interest. Chapter Ten describes how outcomes data can benefit physicians now and in the future. Chapters Eleven and Twelve provide a strategic plan for implementing outcomes measurement in a small practice or a large organization. Chapter Thirteen explains how outcomes data can change physician behavior and improve patient care. Chapter Fourteen tackles the issue of how to market quality in health care services. In Chapter Fifteen Steven Isenberg provides his own practice's experience in using quality data to create competitive advantage. Appendixes A and B provide additional in-depth material on benefit-cost analyses for health care and on developing and interpreting health measures, respectively.

Profiting from Quality: Outcomes Strategies for Medical Practice will provide readers with an understanding of the value of quality in health care and strategies for implementing measurement to improve care and even to achieve competitive advantage. Ultimately both physicians and their patients will profit from quality.

Acknowledgments

We acknowledge the reviewing efforts of Joseph F. Kasper and the editing efforts of Laurie I. Gelb, who worked tirelessly with the team of contributors. We would also like to acknowledge the organizational efforts of Cheryl Davis.

April 1999   Steven F. Isenberg, M.D.
                                                                 Indianapolis

                                                                 Richard E. Gliklich, M.D.
                                                                 Boston

Reference
Ellwood, P. M. "Shattuck Lecture—Outcomes Management: A Technology of Patient Experience." *New England Journal of Medicine,* 1988, *318,* 1549–1556.

The Editors

Steven F. Isenberg M.D. is founder of Project Solo/Physicians Information Exchange, a physician organization that pioneered multisite community-based outcomes research. He is the codirector for the POINT Project for Outcome Sciences, an Internet-based physician outcomes program. He is editor of *Managed Care, Outcomes and Quality: A Practical Guide* (1997) and has written extensively on community-based physician outcomes studies and practice management. He earned his medical degree from Indiana University, where he continues to serve as associate professor.

Richard E. Gliklich M.D. is chairman of Outcome Sciences, a physicians' health outcomes organization. He is founder of the Clinical Outcomes Research Unit of the Massachusetts Eye and Ear Infirmary and an assistant professor at Harvard Medical School. He is a former Charles A. Dana Scholar in Health Services and Outcomes Research. He has an international reputation in outcomes research and related technologies, and his work has been published in over seventy journal articles and book chapters. He holds a B.A. from Yale University and an M.D. from Harvard Medical School.

The Contributors

Joseph T. Branca is a data management consultant with Outcome Sciences, an Internet-based outcomes research organization, where he designs and manages clinical databases and data warehouses. Previously he was research coordinator of the Clinical Outcomes Research Unit at the Massachusetts Eye and Ear Infirmary, a Harvard-affiliated teaching hospital where he had extensive experience coordinating data management for multicenter outcomes studies. He received his undergraduate degree from Amherst College.

May Tsung-mei Cheng is the host of International Forum, a Princeton University-based television program devoted to topics in international trade and finance, national economics, and social policy, including health economics and policy. A native of China, she was raised and educated in Taiwan, where she received a law degree from the National Taiwan University. She completed her graduate training at Yale University, where she received an M.A. in international relations from the Center for International and Area Studies. She has worked for the New Jersey Department of Institutions and Agencies and the Educational Testing Service in Princeton. She is also the cofounder of the private Princeton Junior School.

T. Forcht Dagi is president and managing partner of Cordova Technology Partners, an Atlanta-based venture capital group. In addition to assessing and investing in emerging technologies through his venture fund (particularly those related to health care and the life sciences), he has consulted to medical groups and institutions in strategic planning as well as in marketing and negotiation with managed care organizations. He has also been involved in outcomes research and the study of quality improvement on behalf of professional and regulatory organizations and insurance companies. He

also serves as clinical professor of surgery in the Division of Neu-
rosurgery at the Medical College of Georgia. He holds an A.B.
from Columbia College, an M.D. and M.P.H. from Johns Hopkins
University, an M.T.S. from Harvard University, and an M.B.A. from
the Wharton School of the University of Pennsylvania.

Nancy Peacock Heath has fifteen years' experience in collecting outcomes data and using them to drive physician action. Currently a
consultant with Outcome Sciences, where her work focuses on the
design of outcomes data collection and presentation systems, she
has also developed and implemented outcomes and other programs with a variety of physician groups, including the American
Academy of Orthopaedic Surgeons, the American Association of
Hip and Knee Surgeons, the American Association of Neurologi-
cal Surgeons, and others. She holds a Ph.D. from Purdue University and an undergraduate degree from Yale University.

Megan Morgan has more than ten years' experience in promoting
and developing provider-driven outcomes systems in a number of
health care environments. Well known for her work in organizational strategic planning and patient satisfaction measurement,
she is currently a consultant with Outcome Sciences. She previously managed her own health care and patient satisfaction consulting practice and worked for seven years managing outcomes
initiatives for physician organizations, including the American College of Surgeons.

Uwe E. Reinhardt has taught at Princeton University since 1968. In
1978, he was elected to the Institute of Medicine of the National
Academy of Sciences, on whose governing council he served from
1979 to 1982. He currently serves on the institute's Committee on
Technical Innovation in Medicine and on the Committee on the
Implications of a Physician Surplus. From 1987 to 1990, Reinhardt
was a member of the National Leadership Commission on Healthcare, a private sector initiative established to develop options for
health care reform. He is past president of the Association of
Health Services Research and has served on a number of government committees and commissions. He is currently a member of

the Council on the Economic Impact of Health Reform, a privately funded group of health experts established to track the economic impact of the current revolution in health care delivery and cost control. In 1996, he was appointed to the Board of Health Care Services of the Institute of Medicine, National Academy of Sciences. Reinhardt was or is a member of numerous editorial review boards, among them the *Journal of Health Economics*, the *Milbank Memorial Bank Quarterly*, *Health Affairs*, the *New England Journal of Medicine*, and the *Journal of the American Medical Association*.

Farhan Taghizadeh is a physician, an accomplished programmer, and a software reviewer for an international Web-based medical journal. He recently completed a research year in the Clinical Outcomes Research Unit of the Massachusetts Eye and Ear Infirmary, a Harvard-affiliated teaching hospital. He is currently in postgraduate training at the University of Rochester. Taghizadeh holds an undergraduate degree from Yale University and medical degree from Pennsylvania State University.

Part One

The Economics of Health Care Quality: Theory and Practice

Uwe E. Reinhardt and May Tsung-mei Cheng

Part One explores some of the contentious issues surrounding the quality of health care from an economist's perspective. This exploration of quality has three conceptual components. In Chapter One we argue that a health system has not one but two social objectives: to enhance the quality of life of patients and to enhance the quality of life of those who provide health care. A properly structured health system seeks a reasonable balance between these two objectives. Next, we propose that a high-quality health system does not drive the clinical quality of the treatments it dispenses to its highest possible level; rather, it stops short of that maximum by rationing health care judiciously in an effort to balance the cost of health care with the benefit it produces. Third, we offer the proposition that the overall quality of health care in an entire health system does not necessarily rise with the prices paid for health care. Finally, we question the increasingly popular proposition that the difficult task of assigning money values to health outcomes in the evaluation of health policies can be avoided simply by entrusting the health sector to the "market." Those who favor a free market approach to health care are implicitly proposing that the social value of a particular health service should rise with the wealth of its recipient. That proposition is unlikely to be popular among the general public, once it is properly understood that adoption of free market principles in health care implies this valuation principle.

Chapter Two applies the theories explained in Chapter One. Using empirical evidence, we suggest that no health system today is properly accountable for the quality of the health care it delivers and that none comes close to maximizing the quality of health care for given levels of expenditures, let alone to approximating what economists would call an economically optimal level of quality. Even the generously financed American health system, which prides itself on delivering the best health care in the world, is not immune to this criticism.

We explore at a general level to what extent financial incentives can be used to drive the health system toward optimal levels of quality. Although it is appealing to believe that the financial incentives inherent in health insurance and in methods of paying the providers of health care could be used to guarantee high-quality care, the chapter concludes that financial incentives can at best be facilitating in this regard. It certainly must be the case that antiquated fee schedules (or other payment methods) that do not reflect the cost of applying modern, best clinical practices will build capricious positive and negative income margins into the payments. Such payment methods violate the most fundamental part of the ancient Hippocratic Oath, *Primum non nocere!* (First, do no harm!), because they *will* harm quality directly. They should be brought up-to-date forthwith, in close consultation and negotiation with representatives of physicians and other health care executives who manage the application of clinical practices. But we also conclude that beyond doing no harm, there are limits to what carefully calibrated payment methods in health care can do to ensure good quality.

Ultimately effective quality control in health care requires a careful mix of government regulation and administrative structures within health care facilities themselves. Both need to be supported by compatible payment methods and, even more important, a modern information infrastructure that is yet to be developed anywhere on the globe.

Chapter One

The Quality of Health Care

Uwe E. Reinhardt
May Tsung-mei Cheng

Our nation's health system serves a dual objective: to enhance the quality of life of its clientele by providing that clientele with health care and to enhance the quality of life of the providers of health care, that is, of the doctors, nurses, other health workers, and owners of business establishments who provide the resources used in the production of health care. The system enhances the providers' quality of life by giving them generalized claims on all of the goods and services for sale in the nation—that is, by giving them money. Figure 1.1 illustrates this dual purpose of the health system.

Health care professionals and policy experts often speak of the "resources" available to the health sector. As Figure 1.1 tries to make clear, that is imprecise language, because there are actually two types of resource flows in health care: the *real resource* flow and the *financial resource* flow. Depending on the economic lifestyles among the providers of health care that the rest of society must support with its health spending, a given flow of financial resources can bestow on patients quite different flows of real resources and, by implication, quite different levels of the quality of health care (Reinhardt, 1987). A well-structured health system seeks a proper balance between the two types of quality of life that the system begets. We shall return to this point when we discuss the relationship between the prices paid for health care and its quality.

In freely competitive markets for ordinary commodities, whose attributes can be properly evaluated by the buyers and whose buyers pay the full price out of their own pocket, the

Figure 1.1. Dual Purpose of the Health Care System.

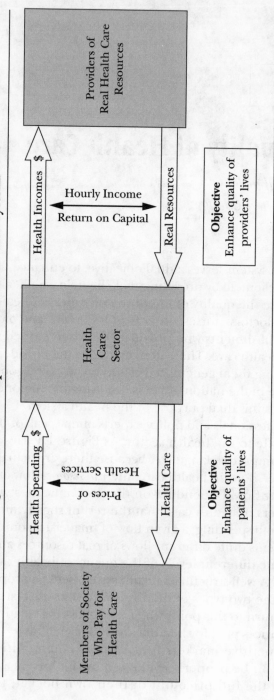

Source: Adapted from Reinhardt (1982). Used with permission of the author.

proper balance between the quality of life of buyers and of sellers is achieved automatically. In such markets a transaction will not take place unless it enhances the quality of life of both parties. Unfortunately that assumption cannot be posited for health care, whose attributes are generally not well understood by patients and which, moreover, typically is paid for by distant health insurers. In that context, enhancements in the quality of life of health care providers can easily come at the direct expense of the quality of life of patients.

This abusive trade-off occurs when patients have been induced to accept medically unnecessary procedures that might have harmed them. It can happen, and is likely to happen, for example, when hospitals base the pay of their staff physicians on the basis of simplistic output measures, such as revenue produced or the number of patients seen or of operations performed per day, without carefully monitoring whether the services rendered were necessary and of acceptable quality. Finally, enhancements in the quality of the providers' life at the expense of patients' lives occur also when the providers of health care use their dominant position in the health care transaction and the powers delegated to them by the state (through licensure) to extract monopolistic profits from the rest of society.[1]

In this chapter we explore the complex linkage that exists between the health care resources purchased by a health system and their impact on the quality of life of the system's clientele, the ultimate manifestation of health care quality.

An Overview: From "Health Care" to "Quality of Life"

Like honor, beauty, and pornography, "quality of health care" is one of those elusive concepts that seem best understood when one does not think too deeply about them. In practice, it is easier to identify gross shortfalls from good quality care than it is to define good quality itself.

Ideally the quality of health care should be measured by the impact it has on the patient's quality of life. Figure 1.2 illustrates the complicated linkages between the health care produced by a health system and the quality of life that system bestows on its clientele (Grossman, 1972; Wagstaff, 1986). The linkage is made up of three interconnected yet distinct production processes: the production of health care, the production of health, and the production of quality of life.

Health Care, Health Capital, and the Quality of Life

First in the linkage is the production process of *health care* itself (box A in Figure 1.2), that is, the health care services rendered by physicians, other health professionals, hospitals and other facilities, the pharmaceutical products prescribed to patients, the services of durable medical equipment patients use, and so on. Figure 1.2 highlights that among the many inputs into the health care production process are the patient's own time and body and, usually, some temporary sacrifice in the patient's quality of life. Misuse of the patient's time—for example, needlessly long waits in waiting rooms, needlessly long hospital stays, and possibly needlessly long absences from work—can substantially raise the true cost of producing health care. Similarly, inadequate management of the patient's pain during and after treatments—allegedly a still common occurrence in modern health care—can be thought of as an avoidable, nonmonetary cost of health care—an input into the production of health care. Alternatively, it could be modeled as an avoidable reduction in the patient's quality of life.

Health care itself, however, is merely one of many inputs into the process that produces *health* (box B in Figure 1.2). Economists think of a person's health as one component of a broader bundle of personal attributes that are lumped together under the generic name of "human capital." The asset "human capital," which includes the knowledge and skills accumulated as part of education and training, is used to earn income, which itself is used to purchase the consumption of goods and services used in the production of what economists call "utility," but is more aptly described as a person's "happiness" or "quality of life" (box C in Figure 1.2). Good health also directly contributes to the individual's ability to convert the consumption of goods and services into a good quality of life—in short, the individual's ability to enjoy life. In Figure 1.2 the arrow running from box B to the circle signals the direct effect labeled "quality of life process."

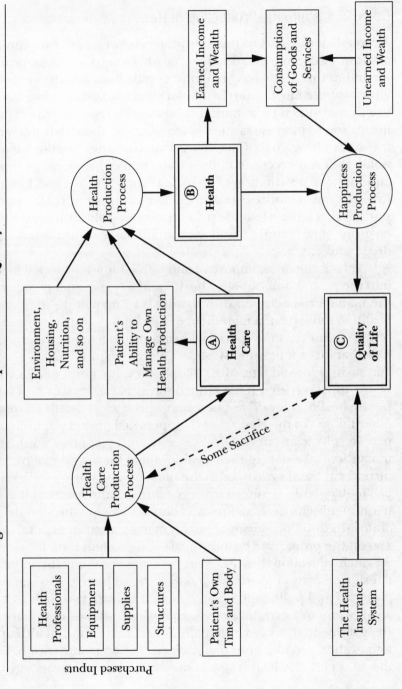

Figure 1.2. Alternative Perspectives on the Quality of Health Care.

Other Inputs into the Production of Health

Although at the level of the individual patient health care can be a matter of the individual's life or death, experts in public health remind us that at the level of entire populations, health care actually is not the most important determinant of population-based health statistics, such as mortality rates or average life expectancy in a nation. If increasing the average scores on these statistics were the overarching goal of health policymakers, most nations today would shift resources out of the production of health care proper and into the production of the other inputs into good health. Among these measures would be better safety measures for transportation, a concerted effort to reduce air pollution and other environmental hazards, and wars on illegal prostitution, illegal drugs, and crime.

Probably the most important and thus far most neglected input into the production of better health and a better quality of life is the managerial acumen of individuals in managing their own health. A fundamental ingredient of that input is the development of a long-run vision on personal health management, that is, the idea that it is a long-run investment decision, just like education and savings for old age. Most people do value good health very highly, especially after it has eroded somewhat. Even so, when people are healthy, they do not necessarily prize good health above all other things. To the chagrin of their personal physicians, ordinary people (physicians in their role as consumers among them) routinely sacrifice a part of their health capital for the sake of higher incomes in the short run or in the pursuit of pleasure—for example, in dangerous leisure activities or through the consumption of harmful substances. A nation can address this issue through deliberate education on personal health management in general and also on the proper use by individuals of the health system.

Such educational efforts must overcome not only the individual's myopia and ignorance, but also the seductive messages of powerful and politically well-connected industries—such as the alcohol and tobacco industries—that spend billions of dollars to steer individuals away from maintaining their good health and toward short-run pleasures that may result in premature death. For the most part, the health system of a country must take as a given the political and advertising power of these merchants of death. It can at most fight these death merchants in the public and political arenas, as the American Medical Association has done recently. Evidently politicians who allow these industries free rein have little interest in the overall health of the population.

To a great extent, the health industry must take as a given the wise or reckless trade-offs that individuals have made in managing their own health. Nevertheless, the health system can affect these trade-offs through the health education that sometimes does and always should accompany the delivery of health care. In Figure 1.2 the ability of health care providers to contribute to their patients' health through this route is indicated by the small arrow running from box A, "health care," to the box that represents the patient's ability to manage his or her own health. Modern breakthroughs in information technology open up entirely new vistas for exploiting this potential.

Finally, aside from health proper, a person's quality of life is affected also by the manner in which health care is financed—roughly speaking, by the nation's health insurance system. The inclusion of a health insurance box in the lower left corner of Figure 1.2 serves as a reminder of that important facet of a health system. At a given level of the quality of health care proper, the quality of life that a health system bestows on individuals depends crucially on whether, after contacting the health system, the individual is driven to despair by incomprehensible insurance claims forms and medical bills or by the prospect of bankruptcy. Incomprehensible bills remain part of the large component of American health care that is still being paid for under the fee-for-service method.

The individual's quality of life depends also on whether the individual needs to worry incessantly about the potential loss of health insurance. For example, the threat of personal bankruptcy over medical bills and a perennial insecurity over the potential loss of job-tied health insurance are permanent features of the American health system. As international surveys reveal, by casting shadows over the purely clinical achievements of the American health care delivery system, America's brittle and chaotic health insurance system detracts considerably from the overall quality of American health care and from the quality of life that Americans enjoy (Blendon and others, 1995).

Defining and Measuring Quality in Health Care

Figure 1.2 makes it clear how difficult it is to develop for practical use a measure of the quality of health care. In principle, such a measure must trace the impact of a particular health care production process through to its ultimate impact on the patient's quality of life. At the moment, that task remains largely intractable. There are just too many intervening variables for which there would have to be statistical control. Furthermore, many of these intervening variables are not even observable.

But here as elsewhere, one should not let perfect become the enemy of good enough. Although the science of defining and measuring quality progresses at its own pace, much headway in practical quality control can be made by ensuring the presence of certain ingredients that are generally thought to be necessary conditions of good-quality health care. Among the many measurable ingredients of this sort are competent health professionals, well-tested and well-maintained equipment, and hygienic health care facilities. Among the necessary ingredients also are processes designed to avoid mishaps during treatment (such as administering improper medication) and also to provide feedback that can support efforts by health professionals at continuous quality improvement (CQI). In many nations, the presence of these ingredients is now monitored through a rigorous process for external accreditation.

Finally, one can approximate the effect of health care on the patient's quality of life by certain crude outcomes-indicators such as infection rates, complication rates, mortality rates, longevity after treatment, the functional and mental status of patients, and the patient's subjective assessments of his or her own quality of life.

The Quality of Health Care: Some Contentious Issues

Figure 1.3 will serve as a framework to highlight certain contentious issues that arise in connection with the quality of health care. In that diagram we are concerned with the contribution that purchased inputs into the production of health care make to the patient's health and, thereby, to the quality of his or her life. In terms of Figure 1.2, the input-output relationship presented in Figure 1.3 includes both the production of health care (box A in Figure 1.2) and the contribution of that health care to the patient's health (box B in Figure 1.2), with all other inputs into the production of health being held constant. (We assume throughout that the nonmonetary cost of the patient's own input into the treatment, including pain and suffering, will be treated as part of the outcome from the treatment.)

On the horizontal axis of Figure 1.3 we plot the money cost of the alternative medical treatments that could be applied to a given illness, arrayed from left to right in increasing order of the costliness of the treatments. On the assumption that the prices of the purchased inputs used in these treatments are fixed, different points on the horizontal axis represent different treatments, although one particular cost figure could conceivably represent two or more distinct medical treatments that all cost the same.

On the vertical axis we represent the maximum contribution to the patient's health that could conceivably be had for the corresponding treatment cost figure on the horizontal axis, given the current state of the art in medicine worldwide. We shall assume that this contribution to the patient's health can be represented by a one-dimensional output index, although that contribution typically is multidimensional, with both positive and negative health effects. We assume that the subjective preference weights used to convert the multidimensional health outcomes from a medical treatment into a one-dimensional output index properly reflect the contribution that these health outcomes make, *on average,* to the quality of life of the typical person in society.

The curved line in Figure 1.3 represents a hypothesized relationship between treatment costs and the maximum feasible value of the one-dimensional output index. Given the structure of Figure 1.3, higher output in this context can also be taken to mean higher quality. We shall therefore refer to this curve as the *cost-quality trade-off frontier* that the health sector faces. If one scaled that one-dimensional quality index so that it is set equal to 100 at its conceivable maximum level, given the current state of the art in medicine worldwide (point C in Figure 1.3), then the degrees of quality that are attained with other medical treatments can be thought of simply as numbers between 0 and 100.

It is reasonable to assume that up to the maximum attainable point where $Q = 100$ (point C in Figure 1.3), increases in the

**Figure 1.3. Cost-Output Trade-off Frontier:
Alternative Treatments for a Given Medical Condition.**

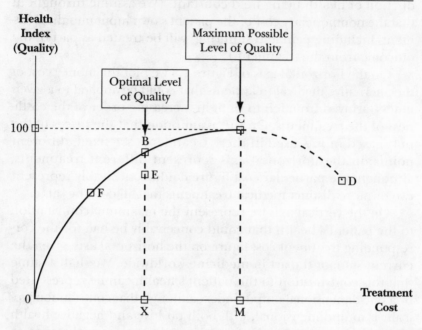

resource intensity and cost of the treatments for a given medical condition produce increased quality. Beyond that theoretical maximum, increases in resource intensity may actually harm the patient's health. They might even kill the patient. Such impairment might occur if the patient were subjected to harmful diagnostic tests, had a pacemaker implanted needlessly, or received dubious but dangerous surgical intervention, such as a coronary artery bypass graft (CABG) that clinical experts would deem unwarranted. It is well known that such overuse of health care does occur in the American health system (Chassin, 1997) and probably in other health systems as well.

Clinical Versus Economic Efficiency

Within the framework sketched out in Figure 1.3, we now distinguish between two types of efficiencies: clinical and economic efficiency.

Clinical Efficiency

A medical treatment is *clinically efficient* if at any given treatment cost level, it maximizes the contribution to the patient's health and minimizes the treatment cost for the contribution it makes to the patient's health. In Figure 1.3 all treatments associated with points on the line segment *OC* are clinically efficient in this sense. Treatments associated with points on line segment *CD* are not, nor are any points below the curve (such as point *E*).

A health system does not need to attain the highest degree of clinical quality to be clinically efficient. Of two countries, the one with a higher observable absolute level of clinical quality than the other may nevertheless be less clinically efficient. (Compare, for example, points *E* and *F* in Figure 1.3.) One should keep that in mind when one compares the typical level of health care quality in, say, the United States, which spends 14 percent of its gross domestic product (GDP) on health care, with the observable level of quality in other nations such as the United Kingdom, which spends only 7 percent of GDP on health care, or in Asia, which spends even smaller percentages of GDP on health care. For all we know, the British National Health Service (NHS) is much more clinically efficient than is the American health system (Klein, 1995).

Clinical *inefficiency* in medical treatments can have several sources. First, the various inputs purchased with the given treatment cost figure on the horizontal axis might be of lower quality than could be had with a more diligent search for inputs of higher quality. For example, the health professionals giving the care might be poorly trained, or their knowledge and skills might have become obsolete even if they had been well educated and trained.

Second, however, even if the inputs going in to medical treatments were of the highest possible quality, the process of using these inputs might be so poorly managed as to lead to inefficiency—to a level of quality below the technically attainable maximum quality for a given treatment cost. (Compare points *E* and *B* in Figure 1.3.) That type of inefficiency is manifest when the use of operating rooms is poorly scheduled, when a hospital observes inadequate hygienic standards or is wasteful in its procurement and use of medical and pharmaceutical supplies, when hospitals and physicians cause iatrogenic disease through the careless administration of drugs (Moore, 1998), or when well-trained health professionals fail to communicate relevant information clearly to patients, at a level that patients can understand.

Finally, clinical inefficiency is manifest when the volume-driven learning effects inherent in complex procedures are not being fully exploited. Research has shown that the mortality and morbidity associated with heart surgery, and often also its costs, is inversely related to the frequency with which a surgeon or a hospital performs the procedure (Chassin, 1997). A recent study of carotid endarterectomy, for example, revealed that "being operated on in a higher-volume hospital conferred a 71 percent reduction in risk for 30-day stroke or death" (Cebul and others, 1998). A failure to concentrate complex and dangerous surgery that is subject to the learning effects in a few centers of excellence can cause serious clinical inefficiency, and it raises profound ethical questions for physicians who perform few of these procedures or perform them at low-volume hospitals. Quite aside from needlessly high treatment costs, that failure can literally lead to avoidable deaths.

The potential of exploiting volume-driven learning effects in health systems tends to be widely disregarded when the hospital sector develops excess capacity and individual hospitals do not or cannot compete on price. This happened in the United States during the 1970s and 1980s, when vast excess capacity developed in the nation's hospital sector and neither privately insured patients nor publicly insured patients, nor their third-party payers, were sensitive to the prices individual hospitals charged. The main competitive instrument left to hospitals was reputation, which they gained through the acquisition of sophisticated technology, in what came to be widely decried as the "medical arms race." Aside from deploring that medical arms race, most policymakers acted helpless in the face of its onslaught. As a result, secondary hospitals began to invade the turf of tertiary hospitals and opened up low-volume heart surgery centers and similar high-tech centers, whose cost and illness-adjusted mortality rates far exceeded those of tertiary centers with higher volumes. Some states sought to control the medical arms race through certificate-of-need (CON) laws, which required a hospital that wanted to open new facilities to demonstrate a need for them in order to obtain permission to put complex new technology in place. When these controls were lifted as part of the general deregulation of American health care during the later 1980s, the cost and mortality associated with heart surgery in the newly decontrolled states rose predictably.

One would think that the pursuit of clinical efficiency in health care at given budget levels for health care should be uncontroversial among the providers of health care, because it does not ask them to sacrifice income. With a given health care budget, the pursuit of clinical efficiency merely requires that the providers of health care do the best for their patients with the incomes that they are already being paid. In principle, that objective should coincide with the provider's own code of ethics. Of course, if the executives of health facilities mistake increases in the number of patient visits per physician hour or the number of surgical operations per physician hour or per operating room hour as "efficiency," then quality-conscious health professionals would and should protest. Unfortunately top managers do lapse from time to time into this mindless notion of "efficiency," thereby visiting great damage on the quality of their institution's output. That mistaken interpretation of efficiency was the chief cause of the shoddy goods and services produced in the centrally planned economies. Quantity of output without adjustment for quality is not only a meaningless yardstick; it is a dangerous yardstick.

Economic Efficiency

To be *economically efficient,* a treatment must be clinically efficient, and it is one such that a further increase in the resource intensity of treatment could not be justified by the "value" of the additional contribution to the patient's health. Point *B* in Figure 1.3, for example, might be that one point on the clinically efficient frontier *OC.* The clinical quality associated with that point falls visibly short of the maximum attainable level, *C.*

To economists, the economically efficient treatment would represent the "best clinical practice" for the medical condition at hand, a judgment that physicians may not accept. Evidently the judgment that the added health outcomes from a more costly treatment do or do not "justify" the added cost of the treatment must be based on some notion of the monetary value of health outcomes. A major question is who should determine that monetary value. We address this important question further on.

An economically efficient treatment would exclude a magnetic resonance image (MRI) or sonogram of a patient, even though the physician believes that these images might have enhanced somewhat the accuracy of the diagnosis and exclude another day in the hospital after surgery, even if there is a small probability that an additional day would have avoided certain complications. Such a treatment might also include a generic drug rather than a more trusted brand-name drug. Some American health insurance companies refuse to pay for a new test to detect cervical cancer that was deemed "significantly more effective" by the U.S. Food and Drug Administration but costs about fifteen to twenty dollars more per test than does the traditional Pap smear (Johannes, 1998). Reportedly one study conducted by a highly respected researcher found that the newer test would cost about $300,000 per additional life-year achieved with it, while the traditional test costs only $27,000 per life-year saved. Evidently such coverage decisions are made purely on grounds of economic efficiency.

It is worth delving into the concepts of clinical and economic efficiency because application of economic efficiency to health care remains controversial among physicians and their patients. As Figure 1.3 clearly indicates, the economist's ideal of "best clinical practices" implies the pervasive rationing of health care, in the sense that potentially beneficial health services are to be denied patients purely for the sake of saving money. Only economists and a few clinicians have defended that proposition explicitly, and probably not even consistently when they themselves are patients (Reinhardt, 1996b).

In the United States, for example, very few managed care companies would state openly that they withhold care for the sake of saving money, because the general public considers the very thought anathema. Along with the physicians who treat and inspire them in this regard, American patients still insist that the optimal medical treatment for a medical condition is that associated with the very top of the cost—quality trade-off frontier (point C in Figure 1.3). The American media and politicians appear to agree.

In any event, the prevailing political posture among politicians, government bureaucrats, and executives of the managed care industry is that only patently useless or harmful procedures will ever be denied patients; in other words, the idea is not to ration health care but merely to rationalize it. In terms of Figure 1.3, rationalizing health care would mean to push the cost trade-off curve as high as it can be and to make sure that no patient ever ends up on the downward-sloping line segment *CD* of the curve. Rationing, on the other hand, would be a retreat from the maximum point *C* toward some lower points *B* or *F* on the curve.

Rationing and the Quality of Care

Figure 1.3 suggests that economic efficiency in health care always must come at the expense of the clinical quality of health care, because an economically efficient resource intensity of medical treatment yields a level of clinical quality (point *B* in Figure 1.3) below the maximum attainable level that could be attained with a more resource-intensive treatment (point *C* in Figure 1.3). That circumstance naturally makes economic efficiency suspect among physicians, who have been trained to and are motivated always to do "the best" for their patients. Yet in his *Clinical Decision-Making* (1996), a collection of essays he had written for physicians and that had been published earlier as a series by the *Journal of the American Medical Association,* physician David Eddy offers a chapter with the seemingly contradictory title "Rationing Resources While Improving Quality." Can "quality" actually be improved through rationing?

The "quality" Eddy has in mind here is not the clinical quality of particular medical treatments, but what he calls the "overall quality" of an entire health system. Eddy imagines a situation in which a defined population must share a fixed pool of real health care resources (health personnel and facilities). The defined population might be a group of people enrolled in a health maintenance organization (HMO), or it may be the citizens of an entire nation covered by a budgeted national health insurance (NHI) scheme, such as Taiwan's, Canada's, or England's. If the budget for the HMO or the NHI scheme is fixed, then with given fee schedules the distribution of access to real health care resources becomes a zero-sum game under which resources used by one group of patients must be denied to another group of patients. With appeal to a number of persuasive examples from daily medical practice, Eddy demonstrates that under fixed real resource budgets, health benefits per dollar spent, as well as the overall quality of care received by the defined population, can be increased by judicious rationing of health care. In his words:

When resources are transferred from practices that have little or no value to practices that have high value, benefits are being transferred from one group of people to another. Each transfer represents a loss of benefit to some, which is a loss of quality, but also represents an increase in benefits to some, which is an increase in quality. To increase overall benefit and overall quality—the quality of care delivered to the entire population—the strategy must ensure that the amount of benefit gained with each transfer is greater, preferably much greater, than the amount of benefit lost [Eddy, 1996, p. 288].

The article on a new test for cervical cancer illustrates a concrete application of this principle. The article reports that many insurers refuse to pay for the more effective but more costly new test on the grounds "that they are better off spending their limited dollars on reminding women [enrolled in their health plans] to get the standard, low-tech [Pap] test regularly" (Johannes, 1998). Presumably they mean by "better off" that their low-tech strategy will save more life-years with a given money budget.

Eddy's proposition is obvious to economists. Yet evidently physicians resist it, so much so that Eddy feels obliged to devote several chapters in his book to this issue. Presumably physicians resist the proposition because as professionals they are trained in an individualist perspective on health care and do not subscribe to the collectivist perspective that drives Eddy's notion of quality.

This gap in perspectives—the individualist perspective of physicians and the collectivist perspective of policymakers—raises a dilemma for physicians and health policymakers alike. If physicians want to take charge of defining the optimal level of quality in health care, then they must necessarily adopt a *collectivist* view. On the other hand, if they prefer to adhere to their *individualist* perspective on quality, then the optimal level of quality, and the resource allocation that goes with it, will be dictated to physicians by nonphysician representatives of society—both legislators and the executives whose institutions directly pay for health services. Physicians should then respect the decisions of these nonphysicians and do the best they can with the resources they are being allocated by the rest of society.

The only apparent escape from this dilemma would be to throw the entire matter into the legendary invisible hand of the free market. It is only an apparent solution, however, because by taking it, one essentially sticks one's head in the sand and lets resource allocation and quality in health care be driven by a distributive ethic that physicians as well as the general public abhor. It is an escape from explicit moral choice. For that reason, most nations do not take it.

National Health Insurance and the Quality of Care

Eddy's collectivist notion of the overall quality produced by a budgeted health system for a defined population remains focused mainly on the quality of medical treatments, but the concept can be extended to other attributes of a nation's health system. It is remarkable, for example, that the American system, which is allocated 14 percent of the nation's GDP and achieves world-class excellence in so many clinical areas, nevertheless earns relatively low marks in international surveys when respondents are asked to rate the quality of the health "system," rather than the quality of the system's "health care."

A broader definition of system's quality would include the purely clinical quality of particular health services and of entire medical treatments, for that is fundamental to good system quality. It would also include the sense of financial security that the health insurance system grants to individuals, the freedom from bureaucratic hassle that it grants to patients and the providers of health care alike, and the sense of fairness that the entire system conveys to the citizenry. It is mainly on these dimensions of overall system quality that the American health system is found wanting by the American public. For lack of a better term, we shall refer to this broad, overall system quality as the *macroquality* of the system and call the purely clinical quality of the medical treatments the system dispenses its *microquality*.

Unless a nation's health system is already excessively endowed with resources, there is likely to be a trade-off between the system's macroquality and microquality. A nation's policymaking elite may decide to emphasize mainly the microquality of the treatments given to those lucky citizens who do have access to such treatments, all the while neglecting other important quality dimensions of the system. This is the approach of American health policy. That policy has stressed the microquality and the physical comfort surrounding the health care for those who can afford that care while accepting severe rationing of health care for the roughly 17 percent of the population who are uninsured at any moment, two-thirds of whom have very modest incomes. This proclivity is manifest also in the current assault in the media and by politicians on the managed care industry. The uproar is over the fact that well-insured Americans might be denied a particular health service for the sake of saving money, even if that form of rationing were demonstrably economically efficient. To withhold health care from insured patients for economic reasons is deemed unacceptable. At the same time, however, not a word is said over the plight of the nation's 44 million or so uninsured.

Other nations consider it important that their health systems be egalitarian, an ethical precept known as the *principle of social solidarity*. These nations are willing to sacrifice for that principle some microquality of care that might otherwise be available to the upper-income classes. They would opt for universal coverage, which they judge morally superior to the quality of an insured person's care. Canada, the European nations, Japan, and Taiwan fall into this group (Campbell and Ikegami, 1998).[2] These nations sometimes limit through government controls the availability of certain high-cost technology (such as imaging or heart surgery) and provide few frills in their health care facilities. In return, they attain a high degree of egalitarianism with their health systems, with overall costs much below the comparable American figures (Andersen, 1997).

It is important to be mindful of these trade-offs among the particular dimensions of a system's quality whenever the topic of universal NHI arises. One evident reason that the policymaking elites in the United States have never embraced universal coverage is that the well-to-do and the well insured have always feared that universal health insurance coverage would either detract from the microquality of their own health care or cost them much more in the form of additional taxes. The American Medical Association, the American Hospital Association, and private insurance carriers have successfully played on that fear in the media and in the political arena, although they oppose NHI because they fear its monopsonistic power and a resulting loss of income.

Nations that have introduced NHI in one major step have experienced trade-offs of this nature. There was such a redistribution of quality in Quebec when it adopted NHI in the 1970s (Enterline, Salter, McDonald, and McDonald, 1973). Shortly after, the utilization of physician services by persons in the lower-income groups increased substantially, at the expense of the higher-income groups, who received fewer visits and experienced an increase in wait time for an appointment with a doctor. There was a similar shift of physician services from higher to lower income groups after the establishment of the British National Health Services (NHS) (Stewart and Enterline, 1961).

In the longer run a nation could try to mitigate the trade-off between micro- and macroquality by adopting a two-tiered health system. There might be one standard of microquality for patients in a tax-financed bottom tier of health care that is available to everyone on equal terms and a higher level of microquality and more luxurious facilities for patients from the upper-income classes who can pay for that quality with their own resources. The acceptance of such a tiered system is purely a political matter. Although two-tiered health systems have some advantages, the upper tier can put inflationary pressure on the bottom tier and thereby make it more difficult to procure high-quality health care for the bottom tier.

Prices and the Quality of Care

We have tacitly assumed that money budgets and the real resource budgets are the same, which is a common posture in discussion on the rationing of health care, but in fact, these two distinct budgets are not at all the same and they serve totally different purposes. Real resources flow to patients; they usually benefit patients, although not always. Money budgets flow to the providers of these real resources and always benefit these providers. The two types of budgets are linked through the money prices that the providers of health care are able to charge per unit of real resource they provide (for example, per hour that they work).

Depending on the prices that the providers of health care charge, two nations that make available to the population the same quantity of real resources per capita may cede to the providers of health care vastly different amounts of GDP per capita as a reward for these real resources. It follows that a nation's total health spending per capita is an unreliable guide to the quantity and quality of the health care bought with that spending. For example, a comparison of expenditures for physicians' services in the United States and Canada found that in 1985, per capita expenditures (in U.S. dollars) for physician services in the United States were 72 percent higher than those in Canada and that these expenditures were "explained entirely by higher fees; the quantity of physicians' services per capita is actually *lower* in the United States than in Canada. U.S. fees for procedures are more than three time as high as Canadian fees; the difference in fees for evaluation and management services is about 80 percent" (Fuchs and Hahn, 1990). Although this study was based on data over a decade old, a more recent analysis of health care received by the elderly in Canada and the United States reached about the same conclusion. The authors conclude that aside from some expensive, high-tech procedures, on balance the elderly in Canada receive *more* physician services than do the American elderly, although Canada overall spends much less on health care per capita than does the United States (Welch, Verilli, Katz, and Latimer, 1996). In 1996, Canadian spending was only about 55 percent of American spending—$2,002 in U.S. dollars per capita in Canada versus $3,708 in the United States—without any deleterious effect on the measurable, overall health status on the Canadian population (Andersen, 1997).

In a detailed comparative study of health spending and the clinical care given in the health systems of the United States, the United Kingdom, and Germany, the international consulting firm McKinsey & Company (1996) also found that although the prices of health care in the United States were about 40 percent higher than they were in Germany, Germans actually received more real health care resources per capita in 1990 than did Americans. Although the authors of the study interpreted this finding as evidence of "lower productivity" in Germany rather than as higher quality of care, evidently the much higher health spending per capita in the United States ($2,439 per capita in the United States versus $1,473 in Germany) did not bestow on Americans a larger quantity of real resources per capita overall. (The authors arrived at this conclusion because the higher real resource use in Germany did not, they believed, lead to a superior clinical outcome as they defined it.)

We note an additional finding in the McKinsey study, because it bears directly on the issue of the overall productivity of an entire health system and on the quality of the health care experiences it produces. According to the study, after all relevant adjustments were made to make the data comparable, Germany was found to spend about $390 more per capita on real medical inputs than did the United States. On the other hand, the United States was found to spend $360 more per capita than did Germany on administration, and another $256 more per capita on a category called "other." In other words, even if the McKinsey team was correct in interpreting the higher German use of medical inputs per capita as lower (clinical) productivity, that productivity gain was more than wiped out by the much higher administrative and other costs of the American health system. As we have already noted, administrative complexity is a major source of discontent with the American health system. In judging the economic merits of fine-tuning a health system—for example, using sophisticated financial incentives such as coinsurance to achieve superior efficiency—other nations should always be mindful, as Americans apparently are not, that resources burned up in administration and other nonclinical activities are added to the cost of health care as well.

Finally, in his 1993 study of health spending and real resources use in several nations, Mark Pauly (1993) concluded, "When politicians and policymakers ask, 'How does Germany (or Canada or the United Kingdom) do it?' a large part of the explanation for a lower GNP share [going to health care] is that they pay health professionals less—not just physicians, but nurses and technologists, too" (p. 158). In other words, relative to the United States, the health systems of these countries cede to the providers of health care fewer generalized claims on GDP per unit of real health care resource (for example, per physician- or nurse-hour). Pauly properly points out that this redistribution of income does not benefit the country as a whole, but it merely is just that: a particular distribution of claims on the GDP between the providers of health care and the rest of society. Economists are not analytically equipped to render value judgments on the distributions of economic privilege among different groups in society. For our purposes we merely note that lower national money budgets for health care need not imply correspondingly lower real resource budgets or a lower quality of health care. It is a simple but important point that must be kept in mind in any discussion on the quality of health care but is often overlooked. Among the providers of health care, it seems widely taken for granted that higher prices for health always go hand in hand with higher quality.

Figure 1.4 illustrates the complex relationship between the price of health care and its quality. The horizontal axis may be thought of as a composite index of the prices paid for health care (P)—a so-called medical care price index. The vertical axis represents a one-dimensional index of quality. It is assumed that a minimum price level X (on the horizontal axis) is necessary just to cover the opportunity costs of the real resources that the providers have relinquished to the process of health care production (including the physicians' own time). If prices do not exceed that threshold level, then in the long run real resources will not flow into health care in the first place. Price increases above X, but only up to level Y on the horizontal axis, are likely to draw increasing quantities of real resources of ever-higher quality into health care and thereby enhance the quality of care. For example, increases in the salary of nurses might draw trained nurses away from currently more lucrative jobs in real estate or in banks and back into nursing care. They might also divert much-needed capital from other industries into the health industry.

But not all price increases are likely to act that way. Beyond a certain level (Y on the horizontal axis) further price increases are likely to enhance merely the quality of life of the providers of health care; they will not add to the quality of the health care that the providers bestow on patients. For example, simply doubling the fee paid to a surgeon for a cataract operation may do nothing at all to enhance the quality of that surgery. It would merely enhance the quality of the surgeon's life. That effect is indicated in Figure 1.5 with the horizontal segment AB of the solid line, which assumes that the health care budget is more or less open-ended, as it was and in many parts of the country still seems to be in the United States. (We leave aside for the moment the loss of disposable income that patients transfer to care providers when the prices of health services rise. That added transfer will, on average, decrease the patient's quality of life because it reduces his or her disposable income.)

On the other hand, if the money budget for health care is more or less fixed, as it is in Taiwan and in many other nations with NHI, then increases in the money prices of health services beyond

Figure 1.4. Effect of Prices on System Quality.

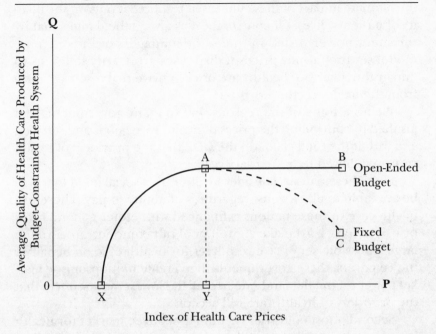

Index of Health Care Prices

level *Y* on the horizontal axis would actually detract from the quality of health care received by patients, because at increased money prices for care, the fixed money budget buys fewer real health care resources. In Figure 1.4 that effect is shown by the downward-sloping dotted line segment *AC*.

The potential of an inverse relationship between the money prices of health care and the quality of health care that can be delivered by an NHI system with a fixed budget is a major reason that so many nations with NHI systems seek to control the prices that they pay for health care through monopoly power on the buying side—through "monopsonistic" power, as economists would put it. They do this by forcing the bulk of health spending to flow through a single budgetary pipe at one point and then control the amount of money that single pipe dispenses per unit of real resource (for example, physician hour) contributed to the health care process. There is evidence that this approach has served to increase at least the quantity of real health care resources available to citizens in many of these nations, although little is known about the ultimate impact of these increased resource inputs on the quality of patients' lives. Of course, there is always the danger that by the sheer power vested in them, the managers of the one-pipe model set the money prices it dispenses arbitrarily so low as to impair the quality of health care or even drive real resources away from the health sector.

We note some of the reasons that so many governments feel justified in controlling the prices of health care goods and services, and with it the total claim on the GDP that the providers of health care are allowed to make every year.

First, these nations consider health care a social good that is to be available to all citizens, regardless of ability to pay. Therefore health care in these nations is financed with either general taxes or payroll taxes. To make a given pool of tax money procure the largest possible set of real resources for health care on behalf of the taxpayers, these governments then create monopsonistic market power on the demand side to seek the lowest money prices that the providers of health care will accept.

Second, most countries do not allow a free market for health services, because they fear that physicians, hospitals, and other providers of health care might exploit financially the ignorance and the anxiety of patients, particularly when patients are severely ill. These nations do not believe that bargains struck between individual health care providers and their anxious patients could ever be fair.[3]

Third, in some of these nations the number of physicians, hospital beds, and pharmacies allowed entry into the health system is artificially restricted, often at the behest of the providers themselves. In the absence of price controls, these artificial limits on supply would bestow undeserved monopoly profits on the providers of health care. Finally, in almost all countries physicians and other health professionals are licensed by government to perform particular health services. As Paul Feldstein (1988) has argued persuasively in his *Health Care Economics,* usually professional licensure is aimed as much or more at protecting the economic turf of particular professions as it is to protect consumers from poor quality. Professions that accept this added monopoly power should expect government to couple it with at least some controls on prices.

For these reasons, many industrialized nations (other than the United States) do not let the prices for health care be determined through bargaining between individual patients and the providers of health care. Instead, government sets these prices (as in Taiwan) or lets them emerge from a process of negotiations between government and associations of providers (as in Canada) or associations of private health insurers and associations of providers (as in Germany). In most nations the negotiated prices are binding on the individual provider of health care. They may not be supplemented by over-the-table side payments (for example, by extra billing of patients) or by under-the-table payments, which are considered professionally unethical and illegal in Canada and in Europe.

Reductions in Prices and the Quality of Health Care

Figure 1.4 seems to imply that providers move to the left and right along the horizontal line segment AB shown in that graph, when prices are increasing or decreasing above the threshold level Y (on the horizontal axis in the figure). In an unbudgeted health system such as that of the United States, for example, this would mean that increases in fees above that threshold level Y would not increase the quality of health care. On the other hand, it would also mean that decreases in fees would not reduce the quality of health care either, as long as fees stayed above the threshold level Y on the horizontal axis. That may not be so, however, if the providers of health care develop notions of a "customary and reasonable" level of remuneration and then use every means available to stay at that level.

Figure 1.5 illustrates this income maintenance hypothesis graphically.[4] Although the figure uses physicians as an example, it can be extended to other health professionals and health care facilities that have the discretion to alter the quantity of the real resources that they package into the service for which a payment is specified in the insurer's fee schedule. The hypothesis applies, for example, to a hospital paid by a flat capitation per medical case or by a flat per diem fee.[5] It similarly can be applied to a nursing home that is paid a flat fee per diem.

Suppose initially that physicians had been paid at the level Y and their fees had then risen to the higher level Z on the horizontal axis.

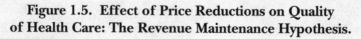

**Figure 1.5. Effect of Price Reductions on Quality
of Health Care: The Revenue Maintenance Hypothesis.**

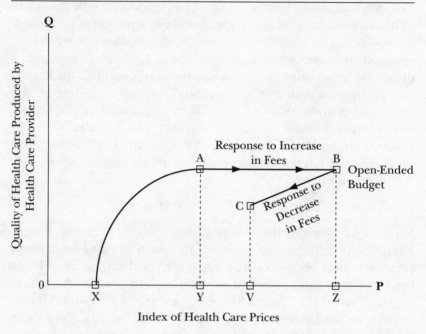

Index of Health Care Prices

As Figure 1.5 is drawn, that increase in fees might not lead to any change in the quality of physician services. It would merely raise physician incomes to a higher level, which would then become the new "customary and reasonable" benchmark for physician income. (Physicians would move to the right along the solid line segment *AB*.) If fees were then judged by the government or by the insurance carrier to be excessive relative to the cost of producing that care,[6] and if fees were therefore reduced to, say, level *V* on the horizontal axis, then physicians probably might not move back along the solid horizontal line segment *AB*. They might not simply learn to live with a lower income for the sake of maintaining the quality of their care at the current level. Instead, physicians might seek to preserve their target income by putting fewer resources into the production of the services for which they now receive the lower fees.

In terms of Figure 1.5, this would mean that physicians would be moving back to the left along the dotted line segment *BC*, not along the flat, solid horizontal line segment *AB*. To do this, physicians might try to maintain their hourly target income by reducing the average length of their patient visits and persuading patients to revisit them more frequently. Physicians might also prescribe more profitable diagnostic tests or procedures that do not require the input of their own time, even if these tests or procedures add little or nothing to the quality of care. In Asian countries, where physicians can profit from selling drugs, physicians also might prescribe more drugs—more than are truly needed and perhaps enough to be inadvertently harmful to patients. Overall these responses might establish practice patterns that deviate substantially from known best practices.

An illustration of this particular income-maintenance hypothesis may have played itself out in the United States in response to cuts in physician fees imposed by private managed care companies.[7] Self-employed American physicians who derive the bulk of their incomes from managed care often complain that the HMOs with which they contract force them to shorten the average length of a visit with patients and thereby reduce the quality of their services. The complaint evokes the image of a direct order by the HMO to physicians not to spend more than *X* minutes per visit with patients. However, few HMOs, other than perhaps a staff model (which employs its own physicians) or a group model (which contracts with one large medical group for physician activities), actually issue such edicts. They would have no reason to do so. Typically an HMO bargains down the fees paid to self-employed physicians for office visits. In response to those drastic fee cuts, physicians then reduce *on their own volition* the average length of their patient visits in order to see more patients per hour and thus maintain their income at the customary level. That is, to be sure, an understandable reaction to a cut in fees. But it is not the HMO that impairs the quality of the physician's care; the physician in the defense of a target income does it.

Target income behavior on the part of providers also might complicate matters in a two-tiered health system, with controlled fees in the tax-financed bottom tier and completely uncontrolled fees in the privately financed upper tier that would be used mainly by well-to-do individuals. One advantage of such a system would be that the powerful moneyed elite in society is more likely to acquiesce in the establishment of a universal, national health insurance system for the lower-income groups, if that elite is not forced to use that universal system and free to purchase for itself another standard of care. Another advantage of such a system is that it offers greater freedom and financing for technical innovation in health care. Third, an upper tier allows the providers of health care to develop high standards for care that is both customer friendly and of high clinical quality.

The willingness and ability of well-to-do patients to pay high fees in the upper tier could raise the income standards that providers consider "reasonable" to very high levels, which would put enormous economic pressure on the bottom tier. The bottom tier, of course, could meet those pressures by raising the prices it pays providers. If its budget were fixed, however, that policy might significantly detract from the quality of its care, because fewer real resources could then be procured with that fixed budget. Severe rationing might ensue. On the other hand, if the bottom tier sought to stretch what it can buy with its fixed budget by keeping the fees it pays low, then it might trigger practice styles that would fall far short of good-quality medicine. In either case, quality in the tax-financed bottom tier would suffer.

Hong Kong currently operates a two-tiered health system of this sort. That system bears close watching, because it can provide practical clues on the effects of two-tiered health care on the cost and quality of health care in the tax-financed bottom tier.

The United States too operated a two-tiered system of this sort for many decades. Until the advent of managed care in the 1990s, the uncontrolled high fees traditionally paid by the private employment-based health insurance system put enormous upward pressure on the tax-financed Medicare system for the elderly and Medicaid system for the poor. To cope with that pressure, the federal Medicare program adapted its fees more or less to the private sector by not letting the average level of its fees slip too much below private sector fees (Physician Payment Review Commission, 1995). To control overall spending, Medicare does not cover many important items—for example, prescription drugs or most long-term care. As a result of this spotty insurance coverage, America's elderly who live at or below the official poverty line still devote over 30 percent of their own meager incomes to health care, in spite of

Medicare (Moon, 1996). By international standards, these American elderly do not enjoy a high-quality overall health care experience, even if the health care that they do receive under Medicare coverage may be of high quality.

For their part, many state-operated Medicaid programs decided to keep fees much below private sector fees. As a result, many providers of health care—notably physicians—refused to treat Medicaid patients at all. These patients often had no other recourse than to turn to so-called Medicaid mills, known to give superficial care of highly dubious quality.

In any event, the complete lack of control over the fees paid by the employment-based, private health insurance tier in the United States (at least until the advent of managed care in the early 1990s) has done great harm to the health care experience of millions of low-income Americans (Reinhardt, 1996a). In addition to the direct economic pressures on the public insurance programs, these high fees probably have served also to price kindness out of the soul of American taxpayers, who are now reluctant even to contemplate the extension of health insurance coverage to all Americans.

Valuing Health and Health Care: Can Free Markets Do It?

Whenever it is said that a particular therapy "is not worth its cost" or is not "economically efficient," a benefit-cost calculus is made that explicitly or implicitly puts a monetary value on the health outcome achieved with the therapy. Noneconomists, particularly physicians, may rightly wonder just how that is to be accomplished in practice—a fair question that has no satisfactory answer so far.

This problem has spawned a huge scholarly literature that remains a source of lively controversy, much of it arising over whose preferences should rule when monetary values are put on health outcomes: physicians, government bureaucrats, insurance executives, healthy people, sick people, social scientists, or someone else.

There has been progress and some consensus on these questions at the conceptual level, and some of the emerging methodology has found application in practice, particularly in the evaluation of pharmaceutical therapies. Here we comment on one simple solution that has gained some popularity around the world recently: that the valuation of health outcomes should be left to the free market, which does such an admirable job in valuing most other commodities produced in democratic societies, from apples to shoes to automobiles. Can the market work its wonders in health care as well?

Some prominent economists and their disciples think so. For example, Milton Friedman (1991) has argued that the ideal health insurance system for a nation would be one in which families have insurance only for catastrophically expensive illnesses, and are required to pay for most other health care out of their own resources, up to an annual, self-paid deductible of $20,000 per year, or 30 percent of the family's annual income, whichever is lower. This idea effectively makes the social value of a particular health service dependent on the recipient's wealth. This is so because free markets follow the famous Roman dictum: *Res tantum valet, quantum vendi potest* (A thing is worth what you can sell it for). This ancient valuation principle is often called the willingness-to-pay principle.

To illustrate the application of this valuation principle to health care, imagine two families, the wealthy Chang family and the poor Li family. Suppose a baby had just been born into each family, and that the Chang baby is healthy, and the Li baby is sickly. According to Friedman's valuation principle, a well-baby visit to a physician by the healthy (and wealthy) Chang baby most likely would be treated as much more valuable than a visit by the sickly (and poor) Li baby to the same physician, because the Chang family probably would be willing *and able* to pay more for that physician visit than the Li family would *and could,* if these two families had to bid for the visit in the free market. Such an outcome might occur even under an ostensibly egalitarian national health insurance with fixed fee schedules, if that system tolerates a flourishing traffic of side payments to physicians. The point here, however, is that Friedman would consider such an outcome as ethically acceptable and "efficient" (Reinhardt, 1997a, 1997b).

It is not difficult to appreciate why some well-to-do people might like the market approach to health care and the valuation principle it implies. But it is just as easy to understand why that approach is rejected by the majority in virtually all modern societies. Writing on this issue, the well-known British economist Alan Williams (1981) has expressed the dominant sentiment concisely:

The [ideal] benefit measure sought is one, which embodies the ethical principle that any interpersonal comparison of the value of health shall not depend upon the wealth or economic value of the people concerned. This reflects not only the *ostensible* ethic of the medical profession itself, but also the putative political principle on which health services are organized in many countries, and it is one of the major reasons why the provision of health services has not been left to the market [emphasis added; p. 273].

We emphasize *ostensible* to draw attention to the contradictory views that many physicians bring to this issue. On the one hand, most physicians probably would profess horror at the notion that the health (or a life-year) of a poor person should be worth less than the health (or a life-year) of a rich person, if that proposition were explicitly put to a vote at the annual meeting of, say, the American Medical Association. On the other hand, many physicians endorse the free market principles for health care espoused by economists such as Milton Friedman, perhaps without quite realizing what distinct distributive ethic and valuation principles for health care they thereby endorse.

We hasten to add that there is nothing inherently wrong with Friedman's social ethic. It is purely a matter of personal preference—of ideology. As such, one should respect it in any debate on health policy, even if one does not endorse it. Nevertheless, there is something wrong with endorsing mutually contradictory ethical precepts.

In any event, people who advocate or endorse the free market approach to health care should be aware of the valuation principle they would thereby impose on health care, and they should be prepared to defend that principle in a debate.

Notes
1.   There can be little doubt, for example, that Americans have been victims of such abuses. Until the 1990s, both the quantity of health services used and their prices were dictated substantially by the supply side of the health care market, against little or no countervailing power on the demand side. This asymmetry in market power, and the vast excess capacity it begot, ultimately led to average annual increases in health insurance premiums of about 20 percent in the late 1980s. The managed care industry in the United States emerged as society's response to these abuses.

2. Under the heading "Universal Coverage and Egalitarian Access" in its report *National Health Insurance Profile 1998,* the Department of Health of the Executive Yuan, Republic of China, declares that "access to health care in Taiwan is a basic civil right" (p. 6).

3. Hong Kong's health system represents a mixture of philosophies. For the bulk of inpatient care and hospital-based outpatient care, Hong Kong relies on the tightly budgeted national health service model. For the bulk of ambulatory care, it effectively allows a free market based on the principle of laissez-faire, which in this instance means "leave doctors and patients alone to hash out the prices of health care." The term *laissez-faire* should never be confused with *competition.* That much misunderstood French term may also mean to leave a monopoly alone to do as it pleases.

4. We thank Princeton University sophomore Mark Cheng Reinhardt for proposing for this chapter, during a conversation on this topic, the thesis that temporarily excessive fees in health care can do lasting damage and especially for proposing Figure 1.5 and the surrounding subsection. Unwittingly, he was tapping into a large, highly technical, scholarly literature on physician-induced demand for health care. For a recent, illuminating addition to this literature, see Tai-Seale, Rice, and Stearns (1998).

5. In the United States, the Medicare program for the elderly categorizes the services rendered by hospitals into some five hundred distinct, diagnostically related cases and pays the hospital a flat fee per case.

6. In the late 1980s, the Medicare program came to just that conclusion for a number of high-tech procedures, such as imaging services, mammograms, cataract surgery, and heart surgery, and drastically slashed the fees for these procedures.

7. While on average the fees paid by the federal Medicare program for the elderly have been about 65 percent to 70 percent of comparable private sector fees, some private sector HMOs in California unilaterally reduced the fees they paid physicians to levels below Medicare levels.

References

Andersen, G. E. "The United States Still Spends More and Fares Worse on Health Indicators Than Do Most Industrialized Nations." *Health Affairs,* 1997, *16.*

Blendon, R. J., and others. "Who Has the Best Health System? A Second Look." *Health Affairs,* 1995, *14,* 220–243.

Campbell, J. C., and Ikegami, N. *The Art of Balance in Health Policy: Maintaining Japan's Low-Cost, Egalitarian System.* New York: Cambridge University Press, 1998.

Cebul, R. D., and others. "Indications, Outcomes and Provider Volumes for Carotid Endarterectomy." *Journal of the American Medical Association*, Apr. 22–29, 1998, pp. 1282–1287.

Chassin, M. R. "Assessing Strategies for Quality Improvement." *Health Affairs*, 1997, *16*, 151–161.

China, Republic of. Department of Health. *National Health Insurance Profile 1998*. 1998.

Eddy, D. M. *Clinical Decision-Making*. Boston: Jones and Bartlett, 1996.

Enterline, P. E., Salter, V., McDonald, A. D., and McDonald, J. C. "The Distribution of Medical Services Before and After 'Free' Medicare Care—The Quebec Experience." *New England Journal of Medicine*, 1973, *289*, 1174–1178.

Feldstein, P. J. *Health Care Economics*. (3rd ed.) New York: Wiley, 1988.

Friedman, M. "Gammons Law Points to Health Care Solution." *Wall Street Journal*, Nov. 12, 1991, p. A21.

Fuchs, V. R., and Hahn, J. S. "How Does Canada Do It? A Comparison of Expenditures for Physicians' Services in the United States and Canada." *New England Journal of Medicine*, 1990, *233*, 884–890.

Grossman, M. "On the Concept of Health Capital and the Demand for Health." *Journal of Political Economy*, 1972, *80*, 223–225.

Huang, A. T. "Thoughts on Three Years' Bed-Side Experience in Taiwan." Paper presented at the Symposium on Medical Education in Taiwan Under National Health Insurance, Taipei, Taiwan, Feb. 26–28, 1993.

Johannes, L. "A New Pap Test Costs More, But Is It Worth It? Some Think Not." *Wall Street Journal*, Aug. 13, 1998, pp. A1, A6.

Klein, R. "'Big Bang Health Reform'—Does it Work? The Case of Britain." *Milbank Quarterly*, 1995, *73*, 209–237.

McKinsey and Company. *Health and Productivity*. New York: McKinsey and Company, 1996.

Moon, M. *Medicare Now and in the Future*. Washington, D.C.: Urban Institute Press, 1996.

Moore, J. D., Jr. "Deadly Consequences: Study Shows Adverse Drug Reactions Take High Tolls." *Modern Healthcare*, Apr. 20, 1998, p. 12.

Pauly, M. V. "U.S. Health Care Costs: The True Untold Story." *Health Affairs*, 1993, *12*, 152–159.

Physician Payment Review Commission. *Annual Report to the Congress*. Mar. 1995.

Reinhardt, U. E. "Table Manners at the Health-Care Feast." In D. Yaggy and W. G. Anlyan (eds.), *Financing Health Care: Competition Versus Regulation*. Cambridge, Mass.: Ballinger, 1982.

Reinhardt, U. E. "Resource-Allocation in Health Care: The Allocation of Life Styles to Providers." *Milbank Memorial Fund Quarterly*, 1987, *65*, 153–176.

Reinhardt, U. E. "Employer-Based Health Insurance: Rest in Peace." In S. A. Altman and U. E. Reinhardt (eds.), *Strategic Choices for a Changing Health System.* Chicago: Health Administration Press, 1996a.

Reinhardt, U. E. "Rationing Health Care: What It Is, What It Is Not, and Why We Cannot Avoid It." In S. A. Altman and U. E. Reinhardt (eds.), *Strategic Choices for a Changing Health System.* Chicago: Health Administration Press, 1996b.

Reinhardt, U. E. *Accountable Health Care: Is It Compatible with Social Solidarity?* London: Office of Health Economics, 1997a.

Reinhardt, U. E. "Abstracting from Distributional Effects, This Policy Is Efficient." In M. L. Barar, T. E. Getzen, and G. L. Stoddard, *Health, Health Care and Health Economics: Perspectives on Distribution.* New York: Wiley, 1997b.

Rowland, D., Feder, J., and Keenan, P. "Uninsured in America: The Causes and Consequences." In S. H. Altman, U. E. Reinhardt, and A. E. Shields (eds.), *The Future U.S. Healthcare System: Who Will Care for the Uninsured?* Chicago: Health Administration Press, 1997.

Stapleton, S. "Latest Tobacco Marketing Target: Women Overseas." *American Medical News,* Aug. 10, 1998, pp. 20–21.

Stewart, W. S., and Enterline, P. "Effects of the National Health Service on Physician Utilization and Health in England and Wales." *New England Journal of Medicine,* 1961, *265,* 1187–1194.

Tai-Seale, M., Rice, T. H., and Stearns, S. C. "Volume Responses to Medicare Payment Reductions with Multiple Payers: A Test of the McGuire-Pauly Model." *Health Economics,* 1998, *7*(3), 199–219.

Wagstaff, A. "The Demand for Health: Some New Empirical Evidence." *Journal of Health Economics,* 1986, *5,* 195–233.

Welch, W.P.D., Verilli, D., Katz, S. J., and Latimer, E. "A Detailed Comparison of Physician Services for the Elderly in the United States and Canada." *Journal of the American Medical Association,* 1996, *275,* 1410–1416.

Williams, A. "Welfare Economics and Health Status Measurement." In J. van der Gaag and M. Perlman (eds.), *Health, Economics, and Health Economics.* Amsterdam: North-Holland, 1981.

Chapter Two

The Cost-Quality Trade-Off

Uwe E. Reinhardt
May Tsung-mei Cheng

This chapter, with additional detail provided in Appendix A, explores the role of health policy to enhance the quality of health care. But first we move from the level of abstraction in Chapter One to a practical review of modern health systems on the cost-quality trade-off curve. Is there evidence that health systems fall short of the levels of quality that they ought to attain with the resources made available to them? Unfortunately there is.

Probably the United States has done as much as or more than any other industrialized nation to measure, monitor, and ensure the quality of health care, as best as that can be done with the current state of the art in quality measurement. Others have presented glimpses at highly successful local initiatives in this ongoing endeavor (Millenson, 1997). These local success stories, however, are but small skirmishes in the battle against a pervasive problem with the quality of care in the United States. Arnold Millstein, medical director of the Pacific Group on Health (a group of thirty-three major California business enterprises that purchase health insurance on behalf of their employees), has projected that on the basis of the available research the *avoidable* medical care–related deaths in the United States are equivalent to "one 747 crashing every day at O'Hare Airport" (Burton, 1998).

In a recent summary Mark Chassin (1997), one the pioneers of quality assessment in the United States, classified them concisely as "misuse, under use and overuse." In terms of the imagery of Figure 1.3, this disturbing verdict translates into the allegation that the American health system places patients all along the system's cost-quality frontier, including the downward-sloping segment where patients are being hurt by excessive care. Just as often, the system puts medical treatments far below the maximum attainable cost-quality frontier.

By *misuse* Chassin means avoidable complications in diagnosis and surgical and drug therapy, and the failure to concentrate in centers of excellence those complex medical procedures that are subject to a steep learning effect. Evidence for *underuse* of health care in the American health system is presented in a growing literature citing large gaps in preventive care and the management of chronic diseases. Recently Lee N. Newcomer (1998), the chief medical officer of United Health Care (one of the largest managed care companies, with over 1 million enrollees), reported on his company's large study of medical claims records. To the researchers' dismay, the study indicated that fewer than half the patients treated by doctors under contract with this HMO were prescribed essential drugs or diagnostic tests for serious conditions such as heart disease and diabetes. "Mediocre is the best word to describe the clinical performance revealed in these [studied] measures," Newcomer concluded (p. 33). In addition, of course, there is likely to be underuse of health care by the roughly 44 million Americans who at any point in time are found without any health insurance.

Finally, there have been many studies in the United States documenting *overuse* of medical procedures, even very dangerous ones. To quote Chassin (1997), "A large number of studies [in the United States] have documented substantial amounts of overuse across a broad spectrum of health care services, including the use of various medications, diagnostic services, and surgical interventions." He includes a lengthy list of specific studies that support his claim.

The proposition that American patients are distributed all along or below the system's maximum attainable cost-quality frontier is corroborated by data regularly published in the *Dartmouth Atlas of Health Care*. This atlas presents, for each county in the United States, comparable statistics on average health spending per capita, the use of certain health services per capita, ratios of physicians and hospital beds per capita, and so on. For the most part, the data reflect the elderly population insured by the federal Medicare program, because it produces the only database that permits such comparisons in the United States. The atlas, accessible on a web site (www.dartmouth.edu/~atlas/), shows that even after adjustments for intercounty differences in the age, sex, and known health status variables of the population, health spending per elderly American insured by the federal Medicare program still varies by a factor of 2. Because the prices Medicare pays providers for health services rendered the elderly are basically the same across the United States, these geographic variations in spending reflect mainly variations in the use of real resources per capita.

American physicians have not been able to defend these variations in practice patterns with appeal to either the health status of the population to be served, or the quality of the care rendered in the various counties, or any other factors. One is entitled to the view that the therapies used in modern medicine often lack a rigorous scientific basis, a highly disturbing conclusion. Evidently there is much room for improving the quality of modern health care without added spending, and mainly through what has come to be known as evidence-based medicine—using results information to guide treatment.

The fact that the United States has gone so far in exposing candidly the misuse, overuse, and underuse practiced in its health system should not be taken to mean that the American health system is uniquely deficient in this regard. Indeed, recognition of the problem through sustained empirical research is a useful first step in remedying deficiencies in the quality of a health system. The American health system should be praised for having gone further in this regard than probably has any other nation. We doubt that health systems of other nations provide health care of a quality that is uniformly superior to the quality of American health care. Many of them might very well perform worse on that score than does the United States. In their otherwise laudatory recent book on Japan's health system, for example, Campbell and Ikegami (1998) comment on the "paternalistic and arrogant" attitude and a "general disregard for responsibility that can be seen not only at the level of the individual providers, but throughout the Japanese health system." They write, "A classic case of lack of accountability is lax supervision and inspection of hospitals. Regulations about staffing ratios and so forth are not very demanding in Japan, but even those regulations are often not enforced very stringently" (p. 180). They go on to report that hospital inspections are announced a week or two in advance rather than by surprise and that the methods of paying health care providers in Japan are not supportive of high-quality medicine. Although Campbell and Ikegami identify some areas in which the Japanese health system does seem to produce better quality than does the American system (mainly in preventive care), the authors would not argue that the Japanese health system exhibits the meticulous attention to high quality that is observed in many Japanese industries or that the health care it dispenses is superior to American health care.

Financial Incentives and Quality Improvement

Improvement in the quality of a nation's health system might be attempted simply by appealing to the compassion and pride in workmanship said to be deeply inculcated in health care professionals. In the United States, there have been numerous efforts to improve health care quality through voluntary adoptions by health professionals and hospital executives of the process of Continuous Quality Improvement (CQI) used in industrial enterprises (Berwick, 1989; Blumenthal, 1993). In this connection, Chassin (1997) has observed that CQI "has spread slowly, its influence limited mostly to hospitals and it has failed to engage clinicians. . . . Relatively little of this effort has made improvement in health outcomes its principal objective." We find Chassin's comments unduly pessimistic. CQI initiatives have as their objectives either lower costs or better clinical outcomes, and often both. They do have their place in a campaign to improve health care quality.

Be that as it may, a major assault on deficiencies in the quality of care probably will require a judicious mixture of government regulation, administrative controls within health care facilities, and economic incentives, all supported by a vast information infrastructure that is yet to be developed anywhere on the globe. In this section we explore the potential for and limits of financial incentives in quality control, after a brief look at the facet of quality that is to be monitored and controlled.

Outcome Versus Inputs and Process

Every so often one hears the statement that only outcomes ultimately matter in health care, which is meant to imply that research
on health care quality should focus mainly on that facet of the production of health (box B or perhaps even box C in Figure 1.2),
rather than the process of producing health care or the inputs
used by that process. This idea is as sound at the theoretical level
as it is unworkable at the level of practice.

If there were agreement among experts on how to define and
measure the outcomes from medical treatments, then one might be
justified in abstracting from the process and the inputs that produced
these outcomes. One would not worry about these facets any more
than consumers worry about the inputs and production processes
that beget ordinary commodities. But the science of defining and
measuring output in health care is still so rudimentary that exclusive
emphasis on outcomes measurement could actually become a major
barrier to more effective quality control. That strategy would needlessly postpone interim attempts to hold the providers of health care
accountable for their work. As Kathleen N. Lohr (1997), a widely recognized expert on quality measurement in health care, has put it,
"Quality measurement should involve both processes and outcomes
of care; a focus on only one will be a mistake. Today's focus on "outcomes management" [in the United States] will not be the answer to
all of the quality problems likely to arise tomorrow" (p. 24). In this
regard, Lohr follows Donabedian's (1966) classical prescription that
quality control in health care should always focus on all three facets of
health care production: the quality of the inputs used, the quality of
the process used, and, where feasible, the health outcomes produced
with health care—sound advice for health policy in any nation.

Ensuring the quality of the inputs used in the production of
health care includes formal approval by government of drugs and
medical devices, as well as strict periodic inspection and accreditation of the facilities that render health care. This can be done by
government agencies or private entities whose seal of approval is
essential for a health care facility's economic survival. The advantage of private entities is that they are less likely to be subject to
lobbying. But these private accreditors can function properly only
if their own economic survival depends on making rigorous and

objective judgments. In the United States, that tends to be the case, and therefore the private sector approach has worked reasonably well in finance and in health care.[1]

Although the quality of pharmaceutical products and medical devices tends to be vigilantly monitored in most countries, relatively little attention has traditionally been paid, in the United States and elsewhere, to the quality of the human capital used in the production of health care, that is, the competence of health professionals. Aside from some supervision through accreditation of the institutions that educate and train health professionals and a one-time examination of health professionals at the start of their careers, there typically are few mechanisms in place to ensure that health professionals keep abreast of the rapidly advancing state of the art in medicine. No country would tolerate that state of affairs in its aviation industry, yet it is tolerated in health care.

There are basically two ways in which such updating could be ensured. First, all health professionals could be required to undergo strict, periodic reexamination for the purpose of relicensing, just as airline pilots are periodically reexamined. Quite understandably, health professionals find the idea of periodic reexamination nettlesome, if not frightening. That approach might be avoided if there were in place a highly transparent information infrastructure that could hold individual professionals formally accountable for their practices, against established norms, and that would simultaneously feed back to practitioners information about their own performance relative to established best practices. Such an information system would provide the continuous professional education of health professionals. In principle, it could be grafted onto virtually any health system, although it seems most naturally compatible with managed care.

The question arises to what extent the financial flows that accompany the delivery of health care could be enlisted to goad the health system toward improved quality. These financial flows have two facets: the health insurance system and the method by which health care providers are compensated.

Incentives Inherent in Health Insurance

To design a health insurance system whose inherent financial incentives might be conducive to high-quality health care, one must resolve the question how patients in their role as consumers can be enlisted in that process. Economists are divided on this question. Some believe that patients can be and should be the ultimate judge of health care quality. That school of thought favors a health insurance system based on so-called medical savings accounts (MSAs, pretax monies set aside for medical expenses). Others believe that quality control in health care must be left in the hands of trained experts. That school of thought tends to favor more regulatory approaches, ranging from a national health system to the systems of private health care regulation now lumped together under the generic term *managed care.* In what follows, we shall comment mainly on the MSA approach and managed care.

Insurance Through Medical Savings Accounts

The concept of MSAs couples catastrophic health insurance policies with savings accounts that are established, owned, and controlled by the individual for the purpose of meeting health care expenses not covered by the catastrophic insurance policy. Deposits into the MSAs are either tax deductible or supplemented with flat, refundable tax credits per capita. For the poor, the accounts might be supplemented with public subsidies (Pauly and Goodman, 1995). The catastrophic insurance policies coupled with MSAs usually have very high annual deductibles—in the United States, about $2,000 per year for individuals and $4,000 to $5,000 per year for a family.

The central idea behind the MSA concept is that the recipients of health care (or their families) should be forced to make the requisite benefit-cost analysis for all of their own health care, unless annual spending for health care exceeds the high annual deductible. Economist Milton Friedman (1991) has proposed such an approach, although the deductible he proposes is much higher than those found in practice today.

The proponents of MSAs do not assume that every patient is expert enough to judge the quality of all of the health care patients receive. Nor do they assume that patients would want to function as major agents of quality control in all matters of health care. Rather, they assume that patients are competent enough to select their primary care physician, who will act as the patient's faithful consultant and agent in making referrals to specialists, hospitals, and other health care facilities.

Physicians and other health professionals are assumed by the MSA proponents to face powerful economic incentives to keep up to date with advances in medicine. Professional obsolescence of primary care physicians would be obvious to patients themselves, according to the MSA theory, and professional obsolescence of specialists would be obvious to the primary care physicians who act as the patient's agents. To attract patients, all of them would have to keep up with modern medicine at all times.

Finally, it is assumed in MSA theory that none of the providers would exploit the economic conflicts of interest inherent in modern health care. The obvious one is the conflict in traditional, unmanaged fee-for-service medicine, the chief compensation method assumed under the MSA concept. But physicians in modern health systems increasingly invest in for-profit hospitals, imaging centers, other specialist services, rehabilitation facilities, nursing homes, and home care agencies to which they might refer patients. The assumption in MSA theory is that these referrals nevertheless would be made strictly in the pursuit of high-quality care rather than with the instinct of health care capitalists seeking to support their investments. Alternatively, it is assumed in MSA theory that any exploitation by physicians of conflicts of interests soon would be detected, by the patient or someone else.

Critics of MSAs doubt that this approach can ensure high-quality health care. For one, they fear that the financial incentives inherent in MSAs would reinforce a natural myopia that makes consumers forgo cost-effective preventive care or timely intervention at the onset of acute illness, thereby increasing the incidence of catastrophic illness and reducing the patient's overall quality of life. Furthermore, these critics do not believe that competition among practitioners would control the conflict of interest in the fee-for-service system, especially the asymmetry of information that gives the providers of health care such a dominant position in the health care transaction.

Finally, the critics of MSAs point to the famous 80/20 rule in health care, according to which in any modern health system about 20 percent of the population accounts for about 80 percent of all health spending in any given year (Berc and Monheit, 1992). In other words, under MSAs the patient's financial incentive not to overuse health care is confined to only a small fraction of total national health spending. Patients would have little incentive to control the overuse of health care once catastrophic insurance coverage sets in, unless the covered treatments were controlled through managed care.

Empirical research on the process by which patients choose doctors and hospitals is still in its infancy and does not strengthen the case for MSAs. So far, even the legendary savvy American shopper has been found to do much better research on selecting cars and television sets than on picking a physician (Kertesz, 1998).

To illustrate, for almost a decade Pennsylvania has reported annually on mortality rates and total hospital charges associated with coronary artery bypass graft (CABG) in the state. For each hospital and for each heart surgeon, predicted mortality rates are calculated on the basis of the age, sex, and health status on admission of heart surgery patients treated by these surgeons and hospitals. These expected mortality rates are then compared with the actual mortality rates achieved by the surgeons and hospitals. The comparisons are published annually on the front pages of daily newspapers, by name of hospital and name of surgeon. The data are also made widely available in the *Consumer's Guide to Coronary Artery Bypass Graft [CABG] Surgery*. In a recent article on the use that patients who faced heart surgery have made of these data, Schneider and Epstein (1996) found that only 12 percent of these patients were aware of these data, in spite of their wide dissemination through the media. More remarkable still, among those who were aware of the data, almost none used the information in their own decision making. In an earlier article on these data, the authors found that cardiologists and other physicians did not use the data either in making referrals of their patients to cardiac surgeons (Schneider and Epstein, 1996). If neither the patients nor decisions of primary care physicians who make referrals to specialists are influenced by outcomes data, it is not clear whether a free market for health care without health insurance would ever mimic properly the market for ordinary commodities when payment is made for health care.

The MSA approach to health insurance is not popular in countries that place a high value on an egalitarian distribution of health care. By leaning so heavily toward the idea of the free market in health care, the MSA concept implicitly embraces the principle that the value of a health service should depend on the wealth of its recipient. Furthermore, the MSA concept is known to saddle chronically ill persons with a higher financial burden than they would bear under more egalitarian health systems. Even in the United States policymakers and the public alike are still viewing the MSA concept with great suspicion. So far, only a tiny minority of households use that approach. On the other hand, policymakers in some Asian countries (Singapore, the People's Republic of China) seem more attracted to the idea.

Managed Care Insurance

Managed care is based on the premises that patients typically lack the technical expertise to control the quality of their own health care effectively and that the individual physician may not always be sufficiently up to date to assess properly the merits of the treatments he or she recommends. Furthermore, the concept is based on the belief that professional ethics alone cannot be relied on to mitigate the financial incentives inherent in unmanaged fee-for-service medicine to overprescribe health services.

These premises imply that the autonomy that has traditionally been granted the individual physician, and was long thought to be the very foundation of high-quality health care, is actually a barrier to high-quality health care. Instead advocates of managed care believe that the relationship between the individual physician and his or her patients needs to be continuously monitored by outside experts and, when found deficient, micromanaged from without, with appeal to preestablished practice guidelines that have been developed by clinical experts.

To implement this approach, consumers under managed care systems are asked to enroll in competing health plans, each associated with a limited network of doctors, hospitals, and other providers of health care. The practice patterns of each provider in the network are continuously monitored through statistical means, and each provider is held to established clinical practice guidelines by the plan's care managers—usually the plan's medical director and his or her staff. In effect, then, consumers are asked to pick their own private health care regulator (health plan) from a menu of competing private regulators, which will then "manage" (that is, "regulate") the preventive care of consumers when they are healthy and the curative care they receive when they are sick.

Because the advocates of managed care do not view patients as effective managers of their own health care, they would not impose on patients financial incentives not to use health care, as the MSA approach would. For that reason patients under managed care typically pay little, if anything, of the cost of the care they actually use, in part to encourage them to use preventive health care that might help lower the overall long-run cost of maintaining their health.

In theory, at least, such an arrangement would seek to combine features of a competitive market with the idea of a national health service, because every competing health plan would in effect represent a budgeted, self-contained, integrated health service. This integration may take the form of common ownership of facilities or be virtual, through binding service contracts. In practice, of course, the idea would make sense only if it were accompanied by a credible information system that allows consumers to choose wisely among the health plans that would thereafter regulate the consumer's health care. Without careful external monitoring of the plans and the availability of credible performance data, a system of private health care regulation is fraught with danger because it would permit the private regulator to exploit ignorant consumers for the sake of private profit. Such a data system does not yet exist in the United States (Reinhardt, 1999), where the idea has been most widely applied, but it is likely to develop in the decade ahead. New Jersey (1997), for example, already publishes annually a detailed list of performance data on all health plans selling managed care insurance in the state.

Most physicians probably do not have difficulty agreeing that patients typically are not qualified to judge the merits of alternative medical interventions, and the traditional, complete autonomy enjoyed by individual physicians can no longer be justified in the light of the disturbing data on variations in practice styles. The question for physicians is whether anyone other than physicians should ever "manage" their patients' care. In fact, much of the current backlash against managed care in the United States, among both patients and physicians, is directed not at the idea that health care needs to be managed somehow. It is directed instead at the direct intervention of private, *for-profit* health insurance carriers into the doctor-patient relationship. Many physicians probably would have less trouble with the idea of managed care (and the

loss of individual autonomy that implies) if physicians as a group
were paid an annual capitation and then were free as colleagues
to monitor among one another the quality of the treatments they
order as individuals. Patients may well prefer that approach to
managed care as well. It is possible that in the United States, managed care will evolve toward this model in the next few decades
(Reinhardt, 1996). Of course, health plans run by physicians also
would have to be subject to the same rigorous external monitoring and performance reporting that is now being sought for com-
mercially run HMOs.

Payment Methods and the Quality of Care

For ordinary commodities, differences in quality are explicitly
rewarded through commensurate differences in payment. The
level of payment for quality is determined through an iterative
process in which producers seek information through the market
on product attributes that buyers desire and are willing to pay for.
In the end, that process leads to the happy outcome that what buyers pay for a particular quality attribute must cover the cost of producing that level of quality, or producers would stop producing it.
All quality is then adequately paid for, and quality that is not paid
for will not be delivered.

This ideal is not easily applied to health care. For one, the
attributes that patients would reward might not coincide with the
attributes that clinicians would judge more important. Patients, for
example, might value more highly physicians who are forever ready
to meet requests for prescription drugs than they might value
physicians who are conservative in prescribing drugs and tend to
lecture their patients on healthy lifestyles. Similarly patients might
be inclined to reward more generously a hospital that has a luxurious appearance than a more spartan hospital with a much lower
rate of nosocomial infection, of which patients might not be aware.
(American hospitals are unwilling to publish their nosocomial
infection rates because they believe that dissemination of such
information would cause staff not to report such infections.)

Furthermore, the bulk of health care is paid for by third parties on behalf of the ultimate recipients of care. These third-party
payers can have only vague notions of the value that their clients

attach to particular attributes of the care they receive. At be
third-party payment for health care will always remain crude. But
even a crude payment system should observe at least the fundamental principle that society expects from the providers of health
care: *Primum non nocere!* (First, do no harm!).

This basic principle is violated when third-party payers set
prices for particular health services so capriciously, and so low, that
conscientious providers of health care cannot cover the reasonable
cost of producing high-quality treatments unless they resort to sub-
terfuge (such as billing for procedures they did not actually perform). In the long run, dishonorable fee schedules tend to beget
dishonorable conduct among providers of health care. Public or
private insurance carriers that impose on a health system fee schedules of this sort are directly responsible for poor quality and should
be held publicly accountable for that mischief.

In the United States, the fees that the federal Medicare program
pays doctors and hospitals for services rendered the elderly are
explicitly designed to pass this test. Initially the fee schedules for
hospitals were based on the actual, average accounting costs of treating cases categorized into diagnostic related groupings. The fee
schedules for physician services were based on costs estimated by
more sophisticated methods (Hsiao and others, 1988a, 1988b). Subsequently these fee schedules have been adjusted continuously, item
by item, in the light of changing technology and new information
on relative costs, in an ongoing process of negotiations between government and health care providers. The Medicare fee schedules,
however, do not and cannot compensate providers explicitly for
differentials in the quality of their own services. They are based on
estimated relative cost scales, not on relative value scales.

Unfortunately, although capricious fee schedules certainly can
do great harm to the quality of care delivered by a health system,
the obverse is not necessarily the case: sensible fee schedules
designed to support good-quality medicine do not necessarily
beget good quality. For example, suppose that initially the fee for
an extensive evaluation of a new patient had been set so low that
the physician could cover costs and earn an adequate income only
by keeping such visits to five minutes. If now that fee were tripled
or quadrupled, can one assume that without additional oversight,
the physician will then allocate fifteen to twenty minutes to the

...ing his or her income constant? Might physicians
...re to established, low-quality practice norms and
...income?

...)sgrod (1997), chief medical officer of Sutter Medical
... in California (a large, integrated health care system),
... ...red various attempts that his organization has made to
link p...sician compensation to quality. His findings are as illuminating as they are discouraging. He observes correctly that such a
linkage presupposes the availability of a robust, acceptable measurement of quality—so far a dream. He concludes his review,
based on extensive experience in the field, with the following
sobering observation:

> In each of the many kinds of large physician groups, we are still
> struggling to figure out how to reward specific elements of physi-
> cian behavior, and compensation arrangements are complex. . . .
> As a practicing physician, I can look at all of the theories about
> physician compensation and quality and yet understand that to
> some extent the theory is irrelevant to my day-to-day life. . . . Physi-
> cian compensation may affect quality but, more critically, whatever
> compensation method we provide should not interfere with the
> basic values of the profession or our ability to develop positive rela-
> tionships with the persons for whom we are responsible [p. 86].

Unfortunately Osgrod's admonition is more easily offered than
obeyed in practice. Policymakers for years have dreamed of ways
to "take money out of medicine," that is, to invent methods of com-
pensating physicians and hospitals that do not affect the manner
in which they treat patients. It remains the search for the Holy
Grail. Under piece-rate compensation (fee-for-service) providers
face a financial incentive to overserve. Under capitation that shifts
the financial risk of a patient's illness onto the provider, the incentive is to enhance income by underserving the patient. Under full
salary, neither incentive is evident; but one takes one's chances with
the physician's productivity or dedication to quality. There simply
is not an ideal method of paying providers of health care. Each
method has advantages and shortcomings (Reinhardt, 1987).

If fee for service is to remain the main method of paying
providers, a good start in rationalizing the payment system might
be made to bundle the many distinct procedures going into stan-

dard medical cases into one composite service, to the extent that it is technically feasible. (Bundling of services is not technically feasible when the cost per case varies substantially above the average cost for the case. If that is so, a single fee for the case would frequently overpay or underpay the providers, exposing them to undue financial risk.) For each such bundled case, the reasonable average cost of well-established best-practice protocols (including a reasonable, negotiated value of the time of self-employed physicians) should then be estimated. Compensation should be based on these estimated average costs, with due allowance for the outlier cases that are so typical in medicine.

For routine ambulatory patient visits, one should establish categories that vary by the complexity and length of the visit. Under the Medicare fee schedule for physicians, for example, there are fifteen distinct fees that vary by complexity and time spent with patients. Ideally, to be compensated by the insurance carrier, physicians should have patients validate by signature the time that the physician claims to have spent with the patient. (The Medicare program does not now require such a countersignature; it should.)

The alternative to fee-for-service payment would be to reorganize the entire health system into a set of vertically integrated mini–health systems (so-called integrated delivery systems, or IDS) and to pay each an annual capitation for assuming the full financial risk of treating all of the illnesses of the enrolled population. However, such an approach is practical only if the capitation is adjusted for the age, gender, and health status of the enrollee; otherwise an IDS with a reputation for excellence in the treatment of costly diseases (such as AIDS or diabetes) might attract a disproportionate number of such patients without being properly compensated for it. Methods of making such adjustments are still in their infancy.

Finally, capitation makes sense only if the capitation is paid to a larger integrated system rather than to the individual physician. In fact, the National Academy of Social Insurance (1998) in the United States recently recommended that "the full-risk capitation for all health services applied to individual providers [such as a primary care physician] should be prohibited in the Medicare program" because the economic incentive for the individual physician to withhold care from patients under individual capitation is just too powerful to be safe.

Note

1. The companies that rate the bonds issued by private corporations
    and by governments, such as Moody's Investors Services and Stan-
    dard & Poor, are not only privately owned but are for-profit enter-
    prises. They are paid by the very entities whose bonds they rate, but
    are not influenced by these entities, because their economic for-
    tune rests on making accurate risk assessments of these entities.
        In the United States, the private, not-for-profit Joint Commission
    on Accreditation of Healthcare Organizations (JCAHO) and the
    private, not-for-profit National Committee on Quality Assurance
    (NCQA) are two bodies that accredit health care entities. The
    JCAHO accredits mainly hospital-based health care delivery systems.
    The NCQA accredits mainly managed care health insurance plans.

References

Berc, M. L., and Alan C. Monheit, A. C. "The Concentration of Health
    Expenditures: An Update." *Health Affairs,* 1992, *11,* 145–149.
Berwick, D. "Continuous Improvement as an Ideal in Health Care." *New
    England Journal of Medicine,* 1989, *320,* 53–56.
Blumenthal, D. "Total Quality Management and Physicians' Clinical Deci-
    sions." *Journal of the American Medical Association,* 1993, *269,*
    2775–2778.
Burton, T. M. "An HMO Checks Up on Its Doctors and Is Disturbed
    Itself." *Wall Street Journal,* Jul. 8, 1998, p. A8.
Campbell, J. C., and Ikegami, N. *The Art of Balance in Health Policy: Main-
    taining Japan's Low-Cost, Egalitarian System.* New York: Cambridge
    University Press, 1998.
Chassin, M. R. "Assessing Strategies for Quality Improvement." *Health
    Affairs,* 1997, *16,* 151–161.
Donabedian, A. "Evaluating the Quality of Medical Care." *Milbank Memo-
    rial Fund Quarterly,* Jul. 1966, pp. 166–203.
European Forum on Quality Improvement in Health Care. Vienna, Austria, Apr.
    23–25, 1998.
Friedman, M. "Gammons Law Points to Health Care Solution." *Wall Street
    Journal,* Nov. 12, 1991, p. A21.
Hsiao, W. C., and others. *A National Study of Resource-Based Relative Value
    Scales for Physician Services: Final Report to the Health Care Financing
    Administration.* Publication 18-C-98795/1–03. Boston: Harvard
    School of Public Health, 1988a.
Hsiao W. C., and others. "Estimating Physicians' Work for a Resource-
    Based Relative Value Scale." *New England Journal of Medicine,* Sept.
    29, 1988b, pp. 835–841.

Kertesz, L. "Making Sense of Health Plan Data." *Modern Healthcare,* Apr. 20, 1998, pp. 99–106.

Lohr, K. N. "How Do We Measure Quality?" *Health Affairs,* 1997, *16,* 22–25.

Millenson, M. L. *Demanding Medical Excellence.* Chicago: University of Chicago Press, 1997.

National Academy of Social Insurance. *Structuring Medicare Choices: Final Report of the Study Panel on Capitation and Choice.* Washington, D.C., Apr. 1998.

New Jersey. Office of Managed Care. Department of Health and Senior Services. *New Jersey HMOs: Performance Reports.* Trenton, N.J.: State of New Jersey, 1997. [www.state.nj.us/health].

Newcomer, L. N. "Perspective: Physician, Measure Thyself." *Health Affairs,* 1998, *17,* 32–35.

Osgrod, E. S. "Compensation and Quality: A Physician's View." *Health Affairs,* 1997, *16,* 82–86.

Pauly, M. V., and Goodman, J. C. "Tax Credits for Health Insurance and Medical Savings Accounts." *Health Affairs,* 1995, *14,* 125–139.

Reinhardt, U. E. "A Framework for Deliberations on the Compensation of Physicians." *Journal of Medical Practice Management,* 1987, *3,* 85–95.

Reinhardt, U. E. "Will Physicians Take Back Medicine?" *Physician Executive,* 1996, *22,* 10–15.

Reinhardt, U. E. "Consumer Choice Under Private Health-Care Regulation: From Theory to Practice." Paper presented to the Princeton Conference on Re-regulating the American Health Sector, Mar. 1999.

Schneider, E. C., and Epstein, A. M. "Influence of Cardiac-Surgery Performance Reports on Referral Practices and Access to Care." *New England Journal of Medicine,* 1996, *296,* 251–256.

Schneider, E. C., and Epstein, A. M. "Use of Public Performance Reports: A Survey of Patients Undergoing Cardiac Surgery." *Journal of the American Medical Association,* May 27, 1998, pp. 1638–1642.

Part Two

Outcomes Measurement and Management: Theory and Practice

Richard E. Gliklich

The goal of this section is to provide a primer in the "outcome sciences." In Chapter Three, a framework for health measurement, management, and improvement is developed that puts the key outcomes concepts into context. Moving from the theoretical to the practical, Chapter Four addresses the clinical research principles involved in designing an outcomes study, while Chapter Five provides a taxonomy of outcomes measures and a guide for those trying to choose amongst them. Outcomes measures comprise only part of the measurements currently being assessed in health care. In Chapter Six, customer or patient satisfaction rounds out the discussion of measures. This focuses on an interaction or an episode of care in which the patient as consumer is asked to rate what has occurred to him or her rather than to report his or her health and well-being. In Chapter Seven, a typical outcomes initiative is described along with the practical issues that must be addressed.

In the remainder of Part Two, the discussion turns to technology and data management. To be successful, data collection and management must be as unobtrusive and practical as possible in the clinical setting. A series of potentially enabling technologies are discussed, and each is rated as to how it will actually affect outcomes measurement or medical practice. The Internet is given special attention as the technology most likely to succeed in facilitating widespread implementation of outcomes measurement and management activities. Since a goal of outcomes management is to help medicine become more quantitative, data management and warehousing systems and methods will play an increasingly important role in daily medical practice. Chapter Nine provides background for this emerging part of medical practice.

Chapter Three

Principles of Outcomes Management

Richard E. Gliklich

The Institute of Medicine has defined quality in health care as "the degree to which health services for individuals and populations increase the likelihood of desired health outcomes and are consistent with current professional knowledge" (Lohr, 1990). Outcomes assessment has been described as a "technology of patient experience" and outcomes management as a method to "increase the likelihood of desired health outcomes" when the definition of health outcomes includes the perspective of the patient (Ellwood, 1988).

Review of the literature for particular methods of outcomes assessment can be evaluated on the basis of the temporal properties of the measurement. *Retrospective outcomes analysis* examines systems in which data collection has already been performed. For example, in a study by Wennberg and colleagues (1998), investigators used an existing Medicare database to determine the incidence of complications following carotid endarterectomy in several hospital settings. The major limitation of retrospective outcomes data is that analysis is being performed on data not necessarily collected for the investigational purpose. Problems include poor data quality, inability to obtain important outcomes data, and incomplete data, particularly for case mix. Although many statistical strategies are employed to improve data quality and applicability, retrospective data analyses, particularly those based on administrative databases, remain flawed and of limited value (Ray, 1997).

Prospective outcomes analysis, in contrast, follows a structured protocol for which data collection is yet to be performed. As a result, staging and stratification can be more clearly assessed, and outcomes variables, such as patient health status, can be followed over time to report change from a baseline. Prospective outcomes studies can also better control for bias and confounding inherent in observational databases through more specific staging and comorbidity stratification. Prospective outcomes data collection through structured collection protocols provides an opportunity to produce more sensitive and precise measurements. In describing outcomes measurement, this book is focused on prospective methodologies.

Components of Outcomes Management Systems

Outcomes measurement systems have three major elements, shown in Figure 3.1: inputs (staging or stratification, processes (such as intervention, therapy, and pathways), and outputs (outcomes). Outcomes management systems add an analysis and feedback mechanism.

Inputs

The first step in designing condition-focused, prospective outcomes management systems is the development of reliable staging or stratification methods. A useful staging paradigm includes the stage of the disease, which is a set of variables known to have an impact on patient outcome, and the stage of the host or patient, referring to the relevant comorbidities. For example, Boyd and Feinstein (1978) examined several staging approaches to Hodgkin's disease and advocated the system with the highest prognostic value for outcome (survival).

The second part of stratification examines the health of the patient from the perspective of coexisting illnesses that may have an impact on the outcomes to be measured. Although there is extensive literature on staging of comorbidities, only some of the methods are applicable in large-scale longitudinal studies. Two methods that are relatively easy to use assess comorbidities based on their presence or absence and on their severity. Both have been demonstrated to have prognostic importance. Kaplan and Feinstein (1974) proposed a method that generates a score from 0 to 3 based on the most severe single comorbidity a patient has. Charl-

Figure 3.1. Outcomes Measurement and Management Systems.

Outcomes Measurement

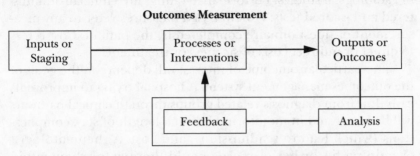

Outcomes Management

son, Pompei, Ales, and MacKenzie (1987) assigned weights to all comorbid diseases to produce a total score. Both methods are reasonably validated and useful.

In addition to staging clinical variables, it is important to collect patient-based and quality-of-life data as part of the initial data collection process. Quality-of-life data are most accurately followed as change from a baseline. In addition, these data may be an important independent predictor for certain health outcomes and therefore should be included as part of the staging data.

Processes

An outcomes management system also measures processes: interventions, medications, personnel, clinical pathways or guidelines, specific procedures, and so on. For many conditions, true end point measurement is not practical or possible, and measurement of process provides the best means to quantify quality of care. When outcomes data are available, cataloguing processes provide the means to determine which processes lead to best outcomes.

Outputs

By defining an end point of interest, one is defining the outcome. A number of outcomes may be of interest for a particular patient or population. Those outcomes fall into broad categories. Traditional measurements include mortality, complication rates, and hospital length of stay. Clinical measures include laboratory tests or radiological studies. Performance ratings are clinician-administered and -scored tests. Patient-based measures refer to any measurement or questionnaire completed by the patient. Cost refers to direct or indirect costs of sickness or treatment.

The particular outcome of interest will depend on the goals of the outcomes management system. A hospital trying to improve its cash flow from diagnosis related groups through clinical pathways will be interested in monitoring hospital length of stay, complications (which lead to readmission), and cost. A rheumatologist examining his or her own use of gold therapy for rheumatoid arthritis will be interested in reviewing patient-based measures of quality of life. A diabetes disease management program may be interested in degree of glucose control, long-term complications, quality of life, and mean cost per diagnosis.

Measurement Science

The utility of all of these outcomes measures for various purposes gives outcomes researchers a wealth of end points to measure. What makes outcomes assessment more attractive today than in the past is the science of health measurement itself, which has enabled us to perform these measurements with increasing levels of precision. Health measurement precision is the necessary ingredient for outcomes management and improvement. Until recently, analytic techniques for evaluating outcomes were limited by measures that reflect events that occur infrequently (such as mortality) or have high variability.

The science of health measurement provides a means to obtain a value on every member of the cohort under study and to minimize the variability of each measurement. Patients start at one health status level and move to another. If the true patient outcome is health status end point, then the effect of the disease or the intervention is reflected by the change in health status.

There are many limitations to health measurement. First, absolute health status (other than death) cannot be known. Rather than quantify true health status change, outcomes measurement quantifies change across a limited array of measures. Second, many current health measures are sensitive at the group rather than the individual patient level, although measurement on the group level is considered sufficient to make broad conclusions that improve care (McHorney and Tarlov, 1995).

General and Condition-Specific Health Measurement

A common approach to assessing outcomes is to combine a condition-focused measure with a generic or general health assessment. In general, condition-specific measures are more sensitive for detecting clinical change and therefore provide more precision in differentiating among therapies. Precision is generally defined as a measure that examines both the range of the measurement and the fineness of the scale (Kessler and Mroczek, 1995). The Chronic Sinusitis Survey, for example, demonstrates a larger standardized response mean, or signal-to-noise ratio, than the Medical Outcomes Study SF–36 in patients undergoing surgery for chronic sinusitis (Gliklich and Metson, 1995). On the other hand, general health measures are generic and can be applied across different conditions, thus providing a basis for comparing one health condition to another. Chronic sinusitis can be shown to be similar to chronic obstructive pulmonary disease in terms of the level of fatigue reported by patients (Gliklich and Hilinski, 1995). Also, general health measures can give an indication of potential side effects of therapy that may be affecting an anatomic region or organ system not addressed by the condition-specific measures. A cancer therapeutic agent might have significant success in decreasing local symptoms, but could cause profound fatigue or depressive symptoms that would not be identified without the general health inventory.

What happens to outcomes assessment when various health measures change to different degrees or even in different directions? For example, in cancer therapy, hearing may diminish from the use of certain chemotherapeutic agents, but survival and bodily pain may both improve as a result of the regimen. How do outcomes assessment strategies choose between different end points to determine relevant change?

Making Sense of Measurement

As more and more outcomes studies incorporate more than one measure, it becomes increasingly difficult to use the measurement for outcomes management, particularly when measures may vary in divergent ways. Despite the fact that health is multidimensional, on a practical level some unidimensional indexes are necessary to use health measurement in such activities as care management. We have used three approaches (utility functions, described in Chapter Four, are a fourth method):

- Importance scaling, where patients rate various symptoms or health-related quality-of-life domains on the basis of importance to their own functioning and well-being. Patient importance determines the weighting of the measure in the final index.
- Composite outcome indexes (COI), which are single scores based on expert panel weightings.
- Balanced outcomes scores (BOS), loosely based on the concept of the balanced score card proposed by Robert Kaplan and David Norton (1996) and used as an overall measure to guide businesses toward their goals. The BOS provides an overall measurement of health performance that can be compared from condition to condition and process to process across an organization.

The search for useful composite measures will continue as the health care industry defines its goals for performance. Accurate measurement and summary scores are the key to using health outcomes information to improve care management. The problems of accurately measuring health are not in any way close to resolution. Limitations in the ability to quantify health status and detect change will not be soon overcome. Considerable research is required in the areas of health services assessment and health outcomes statistics to improve the level of precision with which health can be measured. Despite these limitations, health measurement has reached a level of accuracy and precision that allows it to be applied for improving care.

Outcomes Measurement and Current Quality Assessment

The value of health outcomes measurement in improving care can be understood by examining the current process of quality assessment. Utilization review and quality assessment functions in a typical health care setting focus on two approaches to improving care. First, utilization review examines processes to determine whether pathways, guidelines, and best practices are followed and, if not, where variances occur. This can be termed *process measurement*. For example, a health plan has determined that 200,000 vaccinations for diphtheria in its population is the appropriate level of immunization or that 60,000 women over the age of forty should undergo screening mammography in order to meet the recommended standards set by a reputable advisory panel. Quality assurance is then quantified by dividing the number of patients who received guideline-structured care by the number who are eligible (Palmer, 1997). Other questions too are addressed by evaluating processes: assessing accessibility to care, accuracy of data collection by clinicians, appropriate decision making, adequacy of monitoring, and maintenance of health promotion.

A second function of utilization review is to identify bad events, errors, complications, or outliers of care. For example, the utilization review team will look for readmissions or extended lengths of stay. Morbidity and mortality rounds in medical departments will focus on deaths or unexpected complications. The limitation of this approach is that outliers are by definition rare events. As a result, very few data points are available for statistical analysis, so it is difficult to demonstrate statistically significant differences between one process and another without large samples.

Health measurement provides the opportunity to record data points on all patients with a particular condition. If there is enough precision in the measurements to distinguish one patient from another, then the statistical model can harness the power of the full data set (meaning all of the patients, not just outliers). In the simplest model, a cohort of patients begins at a number of stratified starting points and goes to a number of measured end points. In between is a "black box," which could represent a hospital, a health plan, a surgical procedure, a drug therapy, a clinical pathway, or something else. In reality, the black box contains multiple pathways, processes, errors, costs, and so forth. In an outcomes improvement strategy, the contents of the black box are studied and inventoried. The risk-adjusted outcomes information can then be analyzed through regression techniques to find the elements of the black box that contribute in a positive or negative way to the final outcome.

In this way, systems are analyzed to benchmark outcomes and identify processes or therapies that affect outcomes. The next step is to use these data through passive or active feedback to improve care.

Passive Feedback

An outcomes management or improvement system might be used to present to clinicians the range of variations in treatment for a particular condition and the range of outcomes associated with those variations. In general, physicians respond to data feedback (Marciniak and others, 1998). As a result, this approach can be a powerful way to decrease variations in treatment that result in poor outcomes and to identify good variations. Over time, such an outcomes improvement system is analogous to evolution through natural selection. The "fittest" health processes or treatments survive as bad processes gradually diminish in prevalence and good process variations are recognized and adopted by the group as a whole. In the passive model, behavior is changed through feedback and education.

Active Feedback

In the active model, best pathways, processes, or procedures are identified and then rapidly implemented across the practice or organization. For example, a diabetes disease management system might compare two or three clinical pathways against each other, and a conscious organizational or practice decision may be made to standardize one pathway over another. These are both active approaches to outcomes improvement. As C. David Naylor (1998) has pointed out, "What is already very clear is that the quality of medical care can be measurably improved by knowledge-based interventions."

References

Boyd, N. F., and Feinstein, A. R. "Symptoms as an Index of Growth Rates and Prognosis in Hodgkin's Disease." *Clinical and Investigative Medicine,* 1978, *2,* 25.

Charlson, M. E, Pompei, P., Ales, K. L., and MacKenzie C. R. "A New Method of Classifying Prognostic Comorbidity in Longitudinal Studies: Development and Validation." *Journal of Chronic Disease,* 1987, *40*(5), 373–383.

Codman, E. A. "The Product of a Hospital." *Surgery, Gynecology and Obstetrics,* 1912, *18,* 491–496.

Ellwood, P. M. "Shattuck Lecture—Outcomes Management. A Technology of Patient Experience." *New England Journal of Medicine*, 1988, *318*, 1549–1556.

Gliklich, R. E., and Hilinski, J. "Longitudinal Sensitivity of Generic and Specific Quality of Life Measures in Chronic Sinusitis." *Quality of Life Research*, 1995, *4*, 27–32.

Gliklich, R. E., and Metson, R. "The Health Impact of Chronic Sinusitis in Patients Seeking Otolaryngologic Care." *Otolaryngologic Head and Neck Surgery*, 1995, *113*, 104–109.

Kaplan, M. H., and Feinstein, A. R. "The Importance of Classifying Initial Comorbidity in Evaluating the Outcome of Diabetes Mellitus." *Journal of Chronic Disease*, 1974, *27*, 387–404.

Kaplan, R. S., and Norton, D. P. *The Balanced Score Card*. Boston: Harvard Business School Press, 1996.

Kazis, L. E, Callahan, L. F., Meenan, R. F., and Pincus, T. "Health Status Reports in the Care of Patients with Rheumatoid Arthritis." *Journal of Clinical Epidemiology*, 1990, *43*, 1243–1253.

Kessler, R. C., and Mroczek, D. K. "Measuring the Effects of Medical Interventions." *Medical Care*, 1995, *33*(4 Suppl.), AS109–AS119.

Lohr, K. N. (ed.) Medicare: *A Strategy for Quality Assurance* (vol. 1). Washington, D.C.: National Academy Press, 1990.

Marciniak, T. A., and others. "Improving the Quality of Care for Medicare Patients with Acute Myocardial Infarction: Results from the Cooperative Cardiovascular Project." *Journal of the American Medical Association*, 1998, *279*(17), 1351–1357.

McHorney, C. A., and Tarlov, A. R. "Individual Patient Monitoring in Clinical Practice: Are Available Health Status Surveys Adequate?" *Quality of Life Research*, 1995, *4*, 293–306.

Naylor, C. D. "Better Care and Better Outcomes: The Continuing Challenge." *Journal of the American Medical Association*, 1998, *279*(17), 1392–1394.

Palmer, R. H. "Process-Based Measures of Quality: The Need for Detailed Clinical Data in Large Health Care Databases." *Annals of Internal Medicine*, 1997, *127*, 733–738.

Pollack, M. M., Ruttimann, U. E., and Getson, P. R. "Accurate Prediction of the Outcome of Pediatric Intensive Care: A New Quantitative Method." *New England Journal of Medicine*, 1987, *316*, 134–139.

Ray, W. A. "Policy and Program Analysis Using Administrative Databases." *Annals of Internal Medicine*, 1997, *127*, 712–718.

Wennberg, D. E., Lucas, F. L., Birkmeyer, J. D., Bredenberg, C. E., and Fisher, E. S. "Medicare Population: Trial Hospitals, Volume, and Patient Characteristics." *Journal of the American Medical Association*, 1998, *279*, 1278–1281.

Chapter Four

Outcomes Research Design

Richard E. Gliklich

Outcomes assessment requires the application of rigorous clinical research principles to the real-world setting. Outcomes assessment is hypothesis driven. Once a study question has been delineated, the outcomes team must identify an appropriate population, select an adequate sample, and determine an appropriate sample size.

If a clinical trial is an experimental technique for assessing efficacy, then an outcomes study is a discrete or ongoing effort to evaluate effectiveness. When an outcomes study is intended to be ongoing, it can also be called a *registry*. (Table 4.1 compares clinical trials and outcomes studies.) A clinical trial is generally a prospective study comparing an intervention group and a control group; an outcomes study typically lacks randomization or a control group. As a result, the possibilities for introducing bias in criteria selection or analysis are a greater risk in an outcomes study. Therefore, the importance of applying solid research principles to designing outcomes assessment protocols looms that much larger.

Clinical research studies, whether observational or experimental, share a basic structure. From a general population, a sample is selected. Patients in the sample are assigned to either a study group (receives the treatment, exposure, or disease) or a control group. Assessments are then made as to the outcome of interest. In the analysis phase, comparisons are made between the study group and the control group.

The primary difference between a classical clinical trial and an outcomes study is that in the latter, treatment assignment is observed rather than assigned. For outcomes studies, analysis must take into account two potentially unavoidable errors: selection bias

Table 4.1. Clinical Trials and Outcomes Studies: A Comparison.

Clinical Trials	Outcomes Studies/Registries
Prospective experimental	Prospective observational
Controlled through assignment	Controlled through risk adjustment and stratification
Focus on efficacy	Focus on effectiveness and efficiency
Standard for Food and Drug Administration claims	Not standard for Food and Drug Administration claims
Limitations: Constraints of enrollment and cost	Limitations: Bias and confounding

and confounding. *Selection bias* occurs when the study and control groups differ from each other by a factor that may affect outcome. Even if selection bias is excluded, chance distribution of patients may cause differences in risk factors that affect outcome. *Confounding* is the effect of unaccounted variables that have an independent relationship to the outcome. Some types of confounding can be addressed through statistical techniques.

The first step in design is establishing the central question, the primary reason for the group to perform the study. Typically the central question is framed as a hypothesis. For example, in a study of a surgical procedure, one might hypothesize that the surgeons performing the most procedures have better outcomes than those performing the fewest. If the hypothesis is that there is no significant difference, then the study must have adequate statistical power to detect a difference if one truly exists.

Studies may have several secondary questions, such as those related to subgroups or predictor analysis. A critical component to hypothesis generation is that it should occur prior to data collection and review. Data collection must be designed around the study question in order to obtain the right data; data fishing or dredging (the application of data mining and statistical tools without a hypothesis) can introduce both bias and statistical errors (accepting a significant difference when it may not truly be so because of the problem of multiple *t*-tests). Therefore, data analysis should be driven by the original study questions and hypotheses.

An exception to this concept is in studies of the natural history of a disease or a registry. In this case, it is not the intervention but rather baseline factors that will be analyzed for their relationship to outcomes.

Study Type

Once the aims of the study or project have been defined, the appropriate type of study should be selected. Usually more than one study type can be applied to a clinical question. Although outcomes studies generally focus on prospectively collected observational data, for some clinical questions other modalities should be considered.

Case control or *retrospective studies* have the advantage of using collected data. Traditionally case control models have been employed for studying rare diseases. Case control models are an approach to understanding prior association between risk factors and the disease under study. They have the methodological problems of all other retrospective designs, including recall and reporting bias. Despite these limitations, the case control method is a valid study design for rare diseases or for analyzing rare outcomes in a prospective cohort.

The use of administrative databases is a special case of the retrospective model. These studies are inherently limited by poor data quality, lack of concurrent controls, inability to ascertain important study outcomes, and incomplete data on case mix (Ray, 1997). Several methods are used to adjust for these problems. For example, a common design is to compare a specified period prior to a change with outcomes in a similar period after the change. The inherent problem in this design is controlling for prevailing trend changes. For example, a study of length of hospital stay following a surgical procedure in an interrupted time-series analysis might identify a change in length of stay due to generalized increased pressure from health maintenance organizations to decrease inpatient stays rather than an outcome of an internal intervention. A number of methods exist to address these problems, but invariably the value of these studies is limited.

Cohort studies are observational studies designed to identify the consequences of a single exposure or risk factor. They identify individuals for study without knowledge of whether the disease

under study has developed. Cohort studies can identify the etio-
logical effect of a single factor on multiple outcomes. Many outcomes studies can be considered a type of cohort study.

Cross-sectional studies evaluate the characteristic of interest and
the outcome at the same time point. They provide a snapshot of a
disease population and may be hypothesis generating.

Randomized clinical trials differ from these designs in the assignment of patients to treatment and control groups. Random assignment decreases potential bias in treatment assignment but also
tends to produce comparability in both known and unknown risk
factors. Randomized clinical trials are therefore the gold-standard
approach to evaluating pharmaceuticals in a clinical trial. Unfortunately, from a health services research perspective, randomized
clinical trials are limiting. Random assignment also eliminates the
opportunity to study the effect of nonrandom assignment, often a
goal of outcomes studies. Random assignment in highly controlled
clinical trials does not provide the information necessary to understand the actual effectiveness of a clinical treatment.

Bias

Bias is systematic error caused by both conscious and subconscious
factors. In a clinical trial, the patient and, ideally, the investigator
are blinded to the treatment. In an outcomes study, blinding the
investigator or the patient, or both, is rarely possible. Therefore,
one must be vigilant for sources of bias and evaluate data critically
to identify possible suggestive trends in participant reporting, treatment assignment, data collection, and data analysis.

Study Population

The study population is the portion of the population with the
condition under study who meet the eligibility criteria. Defining
the study population enables others to determine the generaliz-
ability of the findings to other populations. Exclusion criteria,
which generally relate to participant safety, must be explained. For
example, an interventional study may exclude patients over a certain age whom some practitioners may feel should not be offered
the intervention for safety reasons. Up-front exclusion of patients

over a particular age will avoid an obvious selection bias during the study period.

Study Sample

Study sample refers to the actual participants in the study. The study sample is nonrandomly selected from the study population. Although most outcomes studies attempt to enroll consecutive patients, participants must agree to enroll. Typically a log of all eligible patients, maintained at the study site, is evaluated to determine which prospective participants were not enrolled and, whenever possible, to determine if they differed from the enrollees in any significant factor or outcome. Also, all studies are limited by their geographic location or practice environment. Therefore, heterogeneity of the sampling sites may be necessary to achieve a reasonable sample of the study population.

Sample Size

The sample size is the estimated number of patients per treatment group required to achieve statistical significance in a clinical study. For dichotomous response variables, such as those that have two discrete responses (as in yes or no), it is the event rates in the intervention and nonintervention groups that are compared. For continuous response variables, it is a comparison of the mean level in the intervention group versus that of the control. Studies with low statistical power are at greater risk in that effective interventions may not be identified.

Sample size calculations are dependent on two factors: significance level and power. *Significance level* is the likelihood that the difference identified between groups is due to chance alone. In general, investigators will accept a one in twenty chance that the results identified as significant in a study are not truly so (also referred to as Type I error, alpha, or false-positive rate). A one in twenty chance is equivalent to a *p*-value of .05.

The *power* of a study is the likelihood that it will show a significant difference between groups if one truly exists. Studies with low power may fail to reject the null hypothesis when in fact it should be rejected. This is also called type II error, beta, or the false-negative result. Power is actually the probability of correctly rejecting the null hypothesis and is therefore 1-beta. It is a function of sample size, alpha, and the true difference between event rates (delta). A standard level of power for a study is 0.80 or 0.90.

Sample size calculations may be one-sided or two-sided depending on whether the investigator is interested in differences in one direction only or in either direction. An example of a two-sided test is evaluating an endoscopic hernia repair versus a traditional repair, where the result may be better or worse. Sample size is a function of the significance level, the power, and the size of the difference in response. As the size of the difference in response decreases, the sample size necessary to discern that difference as statistically significant increases. If the size of the difference is not known, the investigator should choose a delta that would translate to a clinically important difference.

A special statistical problem develops when one chooses to show that there is no significant difference in effectiveness for an accepted therapy versus a new intervention. The new intervention may have fewer side effects or cost less. For example, the endoscopic hernia repair could be substantially shorter than conventional hernia repair and therefore less expensive to perform. Statistically it is not possible to demonstrate complete equivalence. Special techniques have been developed to estimate sample size for this situation and are beyond the scope of this chapter.

Baseline Evaluation

The baseline is the health status of the patient prior to the intervention or observational period. Beyond stratification and risk adjustment, baseline data are critical for health status evaluation because the change in health status is more reliable than its absolute value as an outcome variable (see Chapter Three). In other words, a comparison of mean change in variable x is a more powerful statistical technique than a comparison of mean values at the end of a study. This translates to either a small sample size or a smaller detectable difference between groups under study. (It is variability that reduces the ability to detect real changes.)

Baseline data are also valuable in determining comparability between treatment groups. This is necessary in both nonrandomized and randomized studies. Even in randomized trials, balance between comparison groups cannot be assumed. In nonrandomized studies, it must be carefully analyzed and reported.

Data Integrity

A study is only as good as its data. Routine audits of data by the Food and Drug Administration for clinical trials between 1977 and 1985 revealed a 12 percent rate of serious deficiencies (Shapiro and Charrow, 1985). If one translates this to nonclinical trials, without significant penalties, the risk of poor data quality must increase. The most significant errors in data collection fall into three categories: incomplete data, incorrect data, and variability. Missing or incomplete data are a strong measure of data collection integrity. Although significant, missing data are always identifiable. Incorrect data are more difficult to identify and therefore more difficult to correct.

Several techniques can be used to help minimize the problems of data quality. For example, a well-designed protocol should be well documented with clear definitions, eligibility criteria, and methods so that investigators can apply them in a consistent manner. The use of standardized study forms can decrease errors and variability. Training reinforces consistency in a study. Small pilot pretesting provides useful feedback on either content or ergonomic problems with study forms. Finally, monitoring of critical points in the study implementation, such as form completion, is important to obtain high-quality data.

The most effective tool to ensure data quality is an audit, performed to increase adherence to the study protocol and its documentation. The auditors need to focus on important errors and limit their process to important information. The rate of necessary verification is variable. The need to back up outcomes assessment protocols with the possibility of an audit may be the strongest factor in ensuring data integrity.

References

Ray, W. A. "Policy and Program Analysis Using Administrative Databases." *Annals of Internal Medicine,* 1997, *127,* 712–718.

Shapiro, M. F., and Charrow, R. P. "Scientific Misconduct in Investigational Drug Trials." *New England Journal of Medicine,* 1985, *312,* 731–736.

Chapter Five

Outcomes Measures

Richard E. Gliklich

Central to measuring health are the outcomes measures themselves. Choosing outcomes measures appropriately and using them
efficiently are critical steps in measuring outcomes successfully.
Even more important to medical practitioners is to understand
exactly what is being measured.

Outcomes measures are constructed for different purposes, so
it is critical to the success of an outcomes endeavor that measures
be selected to match a study's intended purpose. In order to make
those determinations, it is important to understand the meaning
of different performance characteristics of health measures and
how those characteristics will affect a study.

Types of Measures

Outcomes measures should be appropriate to the question under
study, and they should be accurate.

Traditional Measures

Traditional outcomes measures have been generally limited to easily measured parameters, such as mortality and complication rates
or lengths of hospital stay. Although they are important for certain
types of analysis (for example, survival in cancer therapy), evaluating these outliers of care is insufficient for attaining the degree of
precision required in outcomes management systems. These traditional measures identify outliers or are limited to those short-term
measures that can be culled from hospital discharge data, such as

mortality and complication rates, or short-term measures that can be deduced from hospital records, such as length of hospital stay.

From a measurement perspective, traditional measures are significantly limited for the purposes of outcomes improvement. Outlier data are limited because they yield measurements on only a portion of the data set. For example, postoperative bleeding after craniotomy requiring reexploration occurs only a few times in every hundred cases. Therefore, only a few data points are available per one hundred patients. The ideal outcomes measure would yield a discrete measurement for every patient. Thus, there would be one hundred discrete data points. Statistically it is more difficult (meaning it requires several-fold more patients) to show a significant difference between 5 percent and 3 percent than between 50 percent and 30 percent. Length of hospital stay is an intermediate outcome of questionable value—generally reflecting guidelines rather than results. To use industrial terminology, traditional measures are closer to a method of inspection than a method of measurement.

Performance Tests

Performance tests refer to those tests of function that have been called objective. They can be divided into those that produce quantified physiologic parameters (for example, blood pressure, glucose, or prostate specific antigen) and those that generate interpretable data (such as the barium swallow). Physiologic tests generally produce data points that can be studied statistically as continuous variables. The reliability of the data element is known and can be taken into account in the analysis. In some conditions, the value of these data is well accepted and may be strongly correlated to overall function (for example, ejection fraction); in others, the correlation of these measurements to function or survival is less clear (such as mean blood pressure and body mass index). Specific physiologic tests are important as predictors or outcomes for specific conditions. That being said, many physiologic tests are neither predictors nor outcomes. Another category of performance tests is one that produces data that must be interpreted, for example, electrocardiograms and most radiological studies.

Any measure that is interpreted or rated inherently contains variability. There are two levels of variability to consider: variability of the recording instrument and variability in the interpretation.

Neither machines nor humans are completely consistent in record-ing data or making interpretations. Unfortunately, statistical mod-els to account for both aspects of variability in these measures are currently limited. In general, reliability is based on measures of agreement for repeat testing for the same rater and between raters.

There are many examples of poor reliability in such perfor-mance measures in the literature. For example, Feinstein and oth-ers (1970) demonstrated a 20 percent variation in second readings of lung pathology specimens by five experienced pathologists. Sim-ilarly, Davies (1958) showed that repeat electrocardiogram read-ings were subject to a 12.5 percent rate of change from one reading to the next with experienced cardiologists.

Overreliance on performance testing for outcomes management is ill advised for two reasons. First, the issues of reliability are not often addressed in data collection. Second, the relationship of these mea-sures to function, well-being, and survival outcomes is unclear in many conditions. For example, although a positive chest x-ray for metastatic cancer to the lungs is predictive of poor one-year survival, a positive chest x-ray for sarcoidosis has neither predictive nor functional cor-relates. Computed tomography scanning in chronic sinusitis is pre-dictive of neither symptoms nor one-year outcome following surgery.

Cost

Cost is an outcome variable of significant importance. Although seemingly straightforward, cost assessment can be an arduous task because cost accounting methods in health care are poor, and direct costs address only part of the equation. Total costs include direct costs of medical-based resources and indirect costs of lost productivity. In addition, direct costs are often obscured by cost shifting. For example, hospital-reported costs of cardiac bypass surgery may fail to take into account the costs of home care or medications. Direct costs seem to be assessable only from the point of view of the payer. However, few payers pay for all of the costs of illness, and therefore these data too may be questioned.

Quality of Life

Quality-of-life measures address issues of functioning and well-being. Kaplan (1990) and others have stated that for most individuals, only two outcomes are important in interpreting a treatment effect: change in life expectancy or survival and the perceived quality of the remaining years of life.

Health-related quality of life (HRQOL) is currently determined in several ways. If one assumes that there is a set number of domains of health that are universal, such as physical functioning, pain, social functioning, and psychological well-being, and a set of nonoverlapping domains that may be particular to certain health conditions, such as eating and swallowing or appearance, then HRQOL can be divided into two sets of domains: generic domains, which address the common spectrum of health domains (such as physical functioning, role functioning, social functioning, psychological functioning, and overall life satisfaction), and condition-specific domains, which address issues of heightened concern for those with a particular illness. Measurement schemes may draw on a variety of methods to assess such domains: single-item questions, domain-specific measurement addressing a single aspect of HRQOL, a health profile that is a single instrument measuring different dimensions of HRQOL, or a battery of instruments assessing both single and multiple domains of HRQOL.

Quality of life can be assessed by the clinician, for example, by using the Karnofsky Performance Scale; however, this leads to issues of bias that may be difficult to control for. An alternative approach to using clinician-rated scales is the use of patient-based questionnaires. Patient-based outcomes instruments are one of the primary tools for monitoring outcomes. Although physicians in particular have a significant distrust of "subjective" data collection, patient-based instruments are based on sound scientific principles.

In reality, the issue is not the objective versus subjective but whether the information can be trusted. The medical history is an example of a subjective measurement, and one that remains the most important diagnostic and predictive tool in the doctor's bag. But what evidence is there that subjective scales can form a basis for measuring health?

In the mid-1800s the field of psychophysics developed as a method to evaluate the way in which people perceive and make judgments about physical phenomenon, such as the length of a line or the intensity of a painful stimulus. The relevant finding of this nineteenth-century research was that humans can make estimates of subjective phenomena and in a very consistent manner.

In the mid-1940s, numerous scaling techniques were applied to subjective measurements including health indexes. One of the most commonly used applications became the sampling techniques pollsters use to predict voting outcomes. The popularity of these measurements increased, especially in the social and psychological fields. As a result, a statistical science centered on survey construction emerged. This discipline is called psychometrics.

By the 1970s, the concepts of psychometrics were being applied to psychological testing methods. Psychometrics presents a framework for assessing the reliability and validity of items or questions in assessing a particular health concept. In the 1980s, these concepts were applied to clinical medicine in a number of studies, including the Health Insurance Experiment and the Medical Outcomes Study (Ware, 1987). Whether an investigator is assessing health status or patient satisfaction, psychometric principles allow him or her to evaluate the stability, reliability, and validity of the questionnaires or instruments. This permits appropriate statistical formulas to be developed to use these measures.

Psychometrics and clinimetrics (a term used for the application of psychometric principles in the clinical setting) opened a new door on health measurement. As HRQOL measures continue to be developed and used, the valuable role that these measures can play in medical practice has become better understood—for example:

- HRQOL is a significant predictor for survival and other outcomes and therefore is an important baseline risk stratification variable.
- Clinical importance may be easier to define in terms of quality of life than through clinical measures for some conditions (chronic diseases in particular).
- In studies of interventions that may not be significantly different from standard therapy, the important and compelling difference for adopting a new health treatment may lie in fewer side effects as evidenced by a more favorable HRQOL profile.

Developing an Outcomes Assessment Instrument

Outlining the process of developing an outcomes assessment instrument is instructive in order to understand the properties of the measures themselves. The design of any question-based or survey style measure encompasses item selection, reliability, validity, and responsiveness testing. These steps are covered more fully in Appendix A.

Choosing an outcomes measure for an evaluation that may require twelve to eighteen months to complete data collection is a daunting task. Outcome measures must be chosen based on their intended purpose. For example, screening measures will have different characteristics than will evaluative measures. The process of choosing measures often leads to the realization that a measure may need to be developed or reengineered to achieve the stated study or project purpose.

Outcomes measures should be selected for a project using standard criteria on the basis of their intended purpose, that is, how they are to be used in the study. This determination requires a careful review of the instrument's performance characteristics, including its reliability, validity, responsiveness, interpretability, comprehensiveness, and burden. These steps are more fully covered in Appendix B. Table 5.1 presents the types of performance characteristics that can be determined for patient-based measures and the questions about those measures that these characteristics answer.

Reliability of an instrument addresses the question of whether the measurement is reproducible. In reality, reliability has at least two definitions. First, reliability can be thought of as consistency, meaning the stability of the measure if it is repeated over and over on an unchanging subject. Second, reliability is the degree to which different items on the same instrument are answered in a similar fashion when the instrument is administered.

Validity addresses the question of whether the instrument measures what it is intended to measure.

Responsiveness is the degree to which the measure is able to detect clinically significant change in the population or the subject. For studies seeking to evaluate a therapy or intervention, for example, responsiveness is often the critical characteristic in choosing an outcomes measure. Studies using insensitive measures run the risk of not detecting clinically important change.

Interpretability is similar to relevance. What does a change in score mean for the particular patient? Is there a way to anchor the measure to something that is clinically meaningful?

Comprehensiveness reflects how complete the instrument is as an overall assessment of the condition.

Table 5.1 Performance Characteristics of Outcome Measures.

Performance Characteristic	Question Addressed
Reliability	Is the measurement reproducible?
Validity	Does it measure what it is intended to?
Interpretability	What does a change in score mean for a patient?
Comprehensiveness	Does the measure encompass all of the relevant health domains associated with the condition under study?
Burden	What amount of time and effort are required to complete the measure?

Burden is what it takes to administer the measure in terms of time and cost. It is also what it takes for the patient to complete the measure in terms of time and inconvenience. Studies that use measures with high administrative burden are expensive. Those that use measures with high respondent burden tend to have lower response rates.

HRQOL measurement must be rooted to clinical significance. One approach to this calibration is to compare HRQOL measures with changes in other parameters for which clinical impact is known. For example, patients may be asked how many points on a particular scale translates to a significant improvement or decline in their opinion. Another approach, used in the Health Insurance Experiment, is to anchor the measurement to actual events. For example, loss of employment was correlated to a −2.3 unit change on a thirty-eight-item multidimensional instrument.

Utility Measures

An alternative approach to addressing HRQOL is through utility measures or preference scaling. Rather than based on psychometric principles, utility scales are derived from economic and decision theory approaches. Utility scores examine a person's preferences and values for specific health states. The single weighted measure, called the *quality-adjusted life-year* (QALY) provides a single summary score representing the net change in the participant's quality of life and duration of life.

In the utility approach, the patient is presented with the risk of death he or she is willing to take in order to improve his or her state of health. This utility is assigned a numerical value from 0.0 (death) to 1.0 (full health). Revicki and Kaplan (1993) have evaluated HRQOL versus utility measures and reached several conclusions. First, although utility measures are useful for determining change that has occurred due to intervention, they do not indicate in which specific domain of health change has occurred. Second, these measures may not be sensitive to small but meaningful changes in clinical status. In general, psychometric and utility-based methods measure different components of health status that may be complementary in some aspects of outcomes research.

Conclusion

Since it is unlikely that for any condition one measure will be sufficient to provide for all possible studies, it seems unwise to choose one measure over another as the standard. Rather, each instrument should be presented with its performance characteristics, and head-to-head studies of measures should be encouraged to delineate better the advantages and disadvantages of each instrument in particular clinical settings. An expanding inventory of available disease-specific measurement systems requires that users understand how to evaluate instruments critically for their advantages and limitations.

References
Davies, L. G. "Observer Variation in Reports of Electrocardiograms." *British Heart Journal,* 1958, *20,* 153–161.
Feinstein, A. R., and others. "Observer Variability in the Histopathologic Diagnosis of Lung Cancer." *American Review of Respiratory Disease,* 1970, *101,* 671–684.
Kaplan, R. M. "Behavior as the Central Outcome in Healthcare." *American Psychologist,* 1990, *45,* 1211–1220.
Revicki, D. A., and Kaplan, R. M. "Relationship Between Psychometric and Utility-Based Approaches to the Measurement of Health-Related Quality of Life." *Quality of Life Research,* 1993, *2,* 477–487.
Ware, J. E. "Standards for Validating Health Measures: Definition and Content." *Journal of Chronic Disease,* 1987, *40,* 473–480.

Chapter Six

Patient Satisfaction

Megan Morgan

Several trends within the health care delivery system have led to an increased interest in measuring patient satisfaction. Greater price competition for the delivery of health care services and the recognition of patients' role in their own care ("Putting a Premium," 1995) have created an environment in which employers, health plans, providers, and regulatory agencies are all listening more carefully to what patients have to say. Insurers have begun to include patient satisfaction ratings as a key component of internal physician profiles, which in turn is linked to physician compensation. Employers and patients are demanding patient satisfaction data to assess the quality of care provided. Proponents of Total Quality Management, pointing out the pivotal role of the patient as one of the primary "customers" within health care, underscore its importance. Both the Joint Commission on Accreditation of Healthcare Organizations (JCAHO) and the National Committee on Quality Assurance (NCQA) include patient satisfaction surveying as a requirement for accreditation.

Despite the growing interest in—and requirement for—valid patient satisfaction data, confusion and skepticism regarding their value and benefit remain prevalent. Nevertheless, within an increasing competitive health care delivery system, satisfying patients is a fundamental requirement for clinical and financial success.

Patient Satisfaction: A Working Definition

Numerous approaches to defining patient satisfaction have appeared within the literature. The one I use here is, "The patient's (or family's) evaluation of the healthcare services delivered" (Cleary and McNeil, 1988, p. 30). Patient satisfaction can also be defined as a technology of patient experience designed to help payers, patients, and providers make the most cost-effective choices. Finally, patient satisfaction is the experience of care that leaves the patient feeling reassured and better able to take responsibility for his or her own health care.

One of the myths surrounding patient satisfaction is that it is intangible and cannot be measured. In reality, the measurement of patient satisfaction is rapidly developing into a science (Turnbull and Hembree, 1996, p. S42). The origin of the myth can be found in part within the subjective nature of satisfaction ratings. Capturing the perspective of the patient is intentionally more subjective, in that the express attempt is to describe a personal evaluation of care, which cannot be known by direct observation (Ware and others, 1983, p. 247). A common criticism is that satisfaction ratings often do not correspond to providers' evaluation of care. Ware and his colleagues (Ware and others, 1983, p. 247) find this discrepancy to be a crucial strength, indicating that patient satisfaction ratings bring new information to the equation that mirrors the realities of care, as well as reflecting the patient's personal preferences and expectations.

Factors Associated with Satisfaction

A number of factors associated with satisfaction have emerged from the research. Ware and others (1983, p. 248) have brought forward a number of dimensions of care shown to influence overall patient satisfaction.

• Communication and interpersonal manner—the way in which providers interact with the patient. Research indicates that a key component of satisfaction is the communication between the physician (and other health care providers) and the patient. In general, patients are most satisfied when communication has the following elements: information, technical and interpersonal competence, partnership building, social conversation, positive rather than negative talk, and is of a longer duration (Nelson, Woods, Brown, Bronkesh, and Gerbarg, 1997, p. 93).

- Technical quality—the competence of providers and their adherence to high standards of diagnosis. Many, if not most, health care professionals assume that the quality of medical care is determined by the technical competence of the provider (Cleary and McNeil, 1988, p. 29). In reality, technical competence is difficult for a patient to assess accurately. The majority of patients take as a given the competence of their providers absent evidence to the contrary.

- Accessibility and convenience—the amount of time and effort it takes to make an appointment, how long the patient is required to wait in the office. and where the office is located. Research has consistently shown that these are major factors in patient satisfaction, and this dimension of satisfaction is one carefully monitored by managed care organizations. Regardless of how excellent the services are that the organization provides, a patient who cannot access them easily will go elsewhere.

- Finances—the factors involved in paying for medical services (for example, fee for service versus HMO or other managed care plans). This element of patient satisfaction is also of great interest to insurers. For example, the NCQA's Health Employee Data and Information Set (HEDIS) 3.0 survey seeks information about the patient's level of satisfaction with reimbursement under his or her health plan (National Committee on Quality Assurance, 1998).

- Efficacy and outcomes—the result of medical care encounters and the helpfulness of providers in improving or maintaining health. The relationship between patients' perceived improvement in health and satisfaction levels is unclear (Cleary and McNeil, 1988, p. 30).

- Continuity of care—although continuity of care can be maintained if a patient sees several providers at the same location, studies have found that seeing the same physician is positively related to patient satisfaction. (Cleary and McNeil, 1988, p. 29).

- Physical environment—the environment in which care is provided (for example, whether the facility is clean and the atmosphere pleasant).

Not all patient satisfaction surveys measure all of these domains, or areas, of concern. Regardless of the level of detail, experts suggest that quality of service, the interpersonal aspects of care, and accessibility and convenience should always be included (Turnbull and Hembree, 1996, p. S43).

Why Measure Patient Satisfaction?

It is helpful to divide the reasons for measuring patient satisfaction into internal and external motivators.

External Reasons for Measuring Patient Satisfaction

Purchasers of health care are beginning to make their decisions on the basis of value, a composite of cost and quality (Anwar and Capko, 1996). The trend toward the creation of "report cards" for public consumption stems from the need to make information available to both consumers and purchasers. Managed care's objective is to provide value as well: quality outcomes and service with economical use of resources (Anwar and Capko, 1996).

Health plans are also concerned about member retention. Patients who are satisfied with their doctors are more likely to stay with their health plan. (Nelson and others, 1997). An organization's ability to present its own satisfaction data may positively influence negotiations with managed care organizations.

Marketing a practice or health care organization has become increasingly more important in a competitive health care environment. Satisfied patients tell others about their experience, creating positive marketing opportunities and increasing patient referrals. More significant, dissatisfied patients talk to other potential patients about how unhappy they are with their health care experience. Their opinions often influence others in deciding which provider or organization to select for their own health care needs.

Finally, both JCAHO and NCQA require patient satisfaction surveying as part of the accreditation process. This regulatory requirement often motivates organizations to begin systematically measuring the satisfaction of their patients.

Internal Reasons for Measuring Patient Satisfaction

The primary internal reasons for measuring patient satisfaction are to assess and find opportunities to improve the quality of care as well as evaluate organizational effectiveness from the perspective of the patient. Organizations seeking to prove and improve the quality of care provided often look to patient satisfaction as a beginning point for data collection. There is substantial justification for this approach.

Total Quality Management (TQM) places the customer at the center of organizational activities. Although the concept of a patient as a customer seems almost abhorrent to many clinicians and TQM jargon is not always helpful, a customer can be defined as anyone who depends on an organization for services (Goonan, 1995). Clearly the patient is one of the primary "customers" of health care delivery systems. Identifying customer (or patient) needs through the systematic collection of data and meeting or exceeding their expectations are critical factors in successfully practicing within the current health care environment.

There are additional persuasive links between patient satisfaction and quality management. Medical diagnosis and treatment depend to a great extent on accurate patient communication and active patient involvement in the treatment process. Monitoring satisfaction may identify opportunities for improvement in the area of physician-patient communication.

Patient compliance increases with higher satisfaction levels as well (Nelson and others, 1997). Increased compliance with treatment recommendations can lead to improved outcomes, an essential goal of efforts to manage quality most cost effectively.

Practical Issues in Measuring Patient Satisfaction

There are some basic principles to apply in developing a patient satisfaction surveying process:

- Use well-validated, standard surveys within the office. This allows an organization to compare its data with large reference groups and increases the acceptability of results to managed care organizations.
- Inform surveyed patients as to why their opinion is an interest, how they were chosen, how the information will be used, and the procedure to be followed. Respondents should be provided an assurance of anonymity (Isenberg, 1997). This

information can be included in a brief cover letter handed
out to the patients with the surveys.

- Give patients the survey to fill out on-site and deposit in a
  sealed, confidential box conveniently located within the
  office. Mailed surveys have a low response rate. Ask patients
  to complete the survey after (rather than before) the visit
  (Isenberg, 1997).
- Patients staying in a practice have a higher level of satisfaction.
  To overcome the positive selection bias, survey new patients
  or those completing a course of therapy if possible (Isenberg,
  1997).
- Consider a newsletter or other announcement to patients
  informing them of changes made as a result of patient survey
  results.
- Resurvey regularly, and particularly after implementing a
  change based on previous survey results.

Patient satisfaction is one of the four outcomes of any treatment intervention. Its routine measurement within practice is also
one of the easiest to implement. Despite criticisms of the softness
of the data collected, research has shown that it is a valuable source
of both the patient's perspective and a valid method of identifying
methods of improvement within the process of care provided.

References

Anwar, R., and Capko, J. "Managed Care Changes the Approach to Marketing." *American Medical News*, 1996, *38*(12).

Cleary, P. D., and McNeil, B. J. "Patient Satisfaction as an Indicator of
Quality of Care." *Inquiry*, 1988, *25*, 25–36.

Goonan, K. J. *The Juran Prescription: Clinical Quality Management*. San Francisco: Jossey-Bass, 1995.

Isenberg, S. *Surviving and Thriving*. Indianapolis: Willowfingers Enterprises, 1997.

National Committee on Quality Assurance. "Health Employee Data
and Information Set (HEDIS) 3.0 Executive Summary." [http://
www.ncqa.org/hedis/30excum.htm]. Jan. 1998.

Nelson, A. M., Wood, S., Brown, S., Bronkesh, S., and Gerbarg, Z. *Improving Patient Satisfaction Now: How to Earn Patient and Payer Loyalty*.
Gaithersburg, Md.: Aspen, 1997.

"Putting a Premium on Patient Satisfaction." *Managed Care,* 1995.

Turnbull, J., and Hembree, W. "Consumer Information, Patient Satisfaction Surveys, and Public Reports." *American Journal of Medical Quality,* Spring 1996, *11,* S42–S45.

Ware, J. E., Jr., Phillips, J., Yody, B. R., and Adamczyk, J. "Assessment Tools: Functional Health Status and Patient Satisfaction." *American Journal of Medical Quality,* Spring 1996, *11,* S50–S53.

Ware, J. E., Snyder, M., Wright, W. R., and Davies, A. "Defining and Measuring Patient Satisfaction with Medical Care." *Evaluation and Program Planning,* 1983, *6,* 247–263.

Zastowny, T., Stratmann, W., Adams, E., and Fox, M. "Patient Satisfaction and Experience with Health Services and Quality of Care." *Quality Management in Health Care,* 1995, *3*(3), 50–61.

Chapter Seven

Outcomes Studies: The Steps

Richard E. Gliklich

An outcomes study (discrete collection period) or an outcomes registry (ongoing collection) is developed and implemented in a systematic way. First, the feasibility of the outcomes registry is evaluated. The needs of the organization or practice are considered, as are its resources. A budget is developed. For a medical practice, it is wise to start with a common procedure or condition so that data are aggregated at a reasonable rate and interest is maintained. For an organization large enough to implement its own outcomes initiative or registry, the next step is to develop an advisory panel, comprising a group of content experts for both the condition and outcomes assessment, who serve as the task force for the project.

Designing the Protocol

The protocol, which will determine the extent and sources of data collection, the inclusion and exclusion criteria, and the initial plans for analysis, is designed according to the concepts discussed in previous chapters. Structured and streamlined data collection is the key to successful outcomes implementation. Study design and careful choosing of staging and outcomes measurements will determine the success of the study. In a multisite study or outcomes registry, recruitment of other physicians requires forethought and planning.

Designing the Data Collection Instruments

Once the protocol has been established, data collection instruments are designed. Since data collection usually includes baseline, process, and short-and long-term clinical and health status out-comes, an understanding of the care delivery process is critical to constructing an ergonomically efficient system. This requires time and motion studies in the clinical setting to determine the most efficient methods for data collection. If information is available in other places, such as in scheduling or billing software, systems should be established to route information efficiently into the out-comes registry data collection. In addition, the most appropriate routes to obtain patient-based information must be carefully thought through. For example, is clinical stability reached after the last physician visit? If so, data must be collected directly from the patient at work or at home. The data collection instruments, particularly those that require physician input, must be streamlined. Data that will not be analyzed, such as comment fields, are best eliminated prior to data collection. A statistician is a critical element of the planning group. What may seem interesting to the research advisory panel must be congruent with the central study questions.

Outcomes studies are real-world investigations and most commonly fail under the burden of data collection. Three minutes of extra data collection in a thirty-patient day translates to ninety lost minutes from a physician's time. The data collection methods must respect the efficiencies of medical practice. The constant question is not, "What else can we collect?" but rather, "What else can we eliminate?"

When the team has determined that the data collection is efficient is the time to prove that it is not. Data collection should be piloted long before the full study enters its own pilot phase. Once data collection has reached an acceptable point, a protocol book is prepared that includes all of the data collection elements, supporting documents, and training manuals. For multisite studies or outcomes registries, a sample application for human studies committees is prepared for institutions or groups that will require them.

Participation

Physician participation is a critical element in an outcomes study or registry. Prospective, structured data collection requires clinical expertise in some parts of the data collection. This is one of the elements that makes this form of outcomes assessment more powerful and accurate than studies performed on retrospective or administrative databases. Physician recruitment should begin early in the process. The advisory panel forms the core of the first group of participants. The study or registry must have something of value to offer the physicians involved to enlist them in the process. Whether that means recruiting colleagues within one's own practice, specialty, or managed care group, the value of participation must be apparent to physicians other than the investigators. From a properly constructed study or registry, physician participants can and should profit from participation in the ways that have been described in other chapters. Incentive changes a perceived burden to a perceived opportunity.

Patient enrollment follows from physician participation. Patients are generally interested in quality and outcomes and are willing to participate in nonburdensome studies, particularly if their physician is supportive of the study. Occasionally patients receive a small payment as an enticement to complete a long set of measures, although this is more the exception than the rule.

Patients are enrolled consecutively in outcomes studies. A log is maintained at each site of all patients who qualify for enrollment and the reasons of those who choose not to participate. This log is important to be certain that all potentially qualified patients are offered enrollment.

Pilot Phase

Once the protocol is in place, the data collection designed, approvals received, and physicians trained, the pilot phase is ready to begin. The pilot phase inevitably reveals significant problems in the design. This should be viewed as a matter of course; a perfect outcomes pilot has never been launched. In fact, if negative feedback is not being received, the pilot sites are not doing their jobs. Data collection methods are reviewed regularly during the pilot to determine inefficiencies or deficiencies. The outcomes task force must be adaptive rather than defensive.

Generalizing the Study

When a set level of performance is consistently achieved by the pilot sites and all changes have been made in the protocol and collection methods, the study is generalized to more physicians, sites, and patients. New problems often arise as the study leaves the early adopters and is generalized; in fact, this is a second pilot phase of sorts. The task force or advisory panel must again be ready to receive criticism and institute change where feasible.

Frequent checking on the data in the database is an excellent way to monitor the study. An electronic data collection approach facilitates this quality assurance function during the study, since data are immediately available. If other methods are used, then a portion of the early data should be entered into the study database to perform these checks for completeness and data integrity.

Data integrity and quality assurance are further safeguarded by audits and interval analysis of the data. The best method for testing the system is with real data. Frequent reports early on in the process will identify problems missed in the pilot phase. Data management and storage are nontrivial issues that must be thought through carefully at the start of every study. (These issues are discussed more fully in Chapter Nine.)

Analysis

A study is only as good as the analysis performed. Analysis is planned at the start of a study, not at the end. A clear understanding of how the data will be analyzed is prerequisite to designing a study that will fulfill that task. In addition, the statistical plan created in advance of the data avoids fishing expeditions that can lead to incorrect conclusions. Outcomes analysis is a specialized statistical discipline, requiring an understanding of methods to control for bias and confounding, as well as an understanding of health measurement and its properties. The analysis should be performed by someone trained in this area.

Results are then reviewed. Conclusions are drawn and new hypotheses generated. Data collection and reporting continue as an ongoing part of the outcomes management system.

Chapter Eight

Enabling Technologies and the Internet

Richard E. Gliklich and Farhan Taghizadeh

Outcomes assessment is a data collection intensive process. Streamlining the process is critical for making outcomes assessment possible as part of routine clinical practice. There are two components to improving data collection efficiency. First, and foremost, structured data collection must be streamlined by design. No enabling technology will circumvent the need for good planning. Each piece of datum collected must be necessary for the measurement and the analysis, and administrative and respondent burden must be minimized. Improvements in measurement science will help decrease burden. Second, additional improvements in data collection efficiency will come from the enabling technologies, which have been critical in allowing outcomes management to be feasible on a large scale.

Choosing from myriad systems can be difficult, and mistakes can be costly. Essentially the systems can be sorted by the point in the data collection process that they help or replace. Every system must be judged against the standard: pen and paper. Table 8.1 looks at the advantages and limitations of the most common enabling technologies.

A typical outcomes measurement system will include at least three information gathering points:

1. Initial form: Demographic and socioeconomic patient information, clinical staging and comorbidities, and baseline health

Table 8.1. Advantages and
Limitations of Enabling Technologies.

Technology	Advantages	Limitations
Scannable forms	Decrease data entry	Still paper based
Fax servers	Decrease data entry	Telephone charges
Electronic medical records	Data in electronic form	Still developing; inconsistent data dictionaries, integration problems
Mobile devices	Decreases paper, point of care	Extends other systems; does not improve them
Touch screens	Direct patient entry	Useful only in clinical settings
Interactive voice recognition	Decreases paper; leverages telephone	Limited for extended surveys
Internet	Realtime, ubiquitous access	Still developing; does not solve data entry issues

status. The patient and clinician complete some information; additional information may be abstracted from the medical record.

2. Procedural or intervention form: A catalogue or description of the process, pathway, procedure, therapy, or other change (or lack thereof) in the normal course of events to which the patient is "exposed." The process is reported by a physician or other clinician, or is catalogued from charts.

3. Outcome form: An end point of interest that may include clinical, laboratory, financial, or patient-based information.

All of the data are then entered into a database developed for the purpose. The process builds in complexity. Staff are needed to check regularly for interval interventions or therapies that patients may have received, often from other providers. Information is typically decentralized in multiple medical records (office and hospital) and other information systems (scheduling and billing). Patient-reported follow-up data must be rigorously tracked, because patients who go elsewhere and are not accounted for will bias the measurement. On a practical level, finding patients and administering surveys are cumbersome tasks, not only because of the time and effort required, but because of the need to maintain patient confidentiality. In a mobile society, the longer the follow-up period needed to reach clinical stability is, the more difficult it is to maintain follow-up. In addition, technologies that decrease either burden or staff needs will improve efficiency. However, every technology must be judged against what it replaces.

The major area for technologically driven resource consolidation in outcomes measurement is in reducing the number of steps from the clinical event or the survey to the database. If paper is never generated, then it never needs to be entered, stored, or discarded. Most important, any part of the system that requires the same data to be entered more than once is a place to improve efficiency.

Scannable Forms and Fax Servers

The first technological advance is in the use of scanning software. Scannable forms do little to change data collection, but in some situations their use may decrease the costs associated with data entry. Scannable forms provide an immediate solution for organizing large amounts of patient survey information. Using software for standard form generation, one can design and print forms that are spaced and organized optimally for scanning. This software also allows for individual form marking, where forms are printed with information on distribution site and time. With low-resolution document production scanners (scanners that quickly scan text), optical character recognition software allows the user to customize it to pick up hand-marked answers on survey forms. This information is marked and the information directly fed into a database. Each survey can also be individually printed to account for a patient identification number that can be scanned along with the survey. All of this information is then programmed to fit into individual data fields in any database format. The scanned survey sheets fit into preset data fields, organized by site, date, and patient. Most current scannable software systems are compatible with several common ODBC-compliant (Open Database Connectivity) databases.

Although scannable forms seem to limit data entry, in reality, a knowledgeable data entry person is required to oversee the process and adjudicate uncertainties when there is poor character recognition or inadequate markings on the forms. The software remains imperfect in recognizing written characters, and humans are imperfect in completing standardized forms. Depending on the size of the database being developed, this may or may not be more cost-effective than standard keypunch data entry.

Optimizing the value of scannable form software is achieved through several approaches. The key factor in maintaining high confidence intervals is proper form design. Free-text hand print scanning provides the lowest level of recognition, even with forms design software providing boxed spaces for each printed letter or number. Although handwriting recognition is adequate for basic demographic data such as name and address, it is inadequate for the actual outcomes data collection. Therefore, it is highly recommended that survey forms be completed with mark-sense forms (that is, bubbles, ovals, responses to be circled) to obtain accurate levels of data scanning. Well-spaced questions are key for mark-sense forms. Finally, as with any other database, preset validation measures, such as ODBC database comparisons, field checks for outlying data, or custom mathematical checking, can and should be entered into the database. Scanning alone does not maintain validity.

Scannable form software provides the capability to expand and accommodate growing form volumes. As paper volume increases, scannable form software makes more sense. Current systems allow for more than two thousand single-sheet forms per day to be processed; this rate can be expanded through networks that grow quickly to accommodate very large volumes. In addition to scanning, the software generally allows programming to direct the inflow into the appropriate database.

The problem with scannable forms is that they do not eliminate paper. For large volumes of data, significant manpower can be required to feed the form scanners. Furthermore, the process of form creation requires training, and if surveys are marked individually with bar codes for tracking, the process grows in complexity. A multisite outcomes registry can create significant paper for storage or destruction and significant costs in mailing. A single clinical site participating in multiple outcomes registries can be overwhelmed by the paper volume alone. Therefore, scannable software should be considered an interim solution, but it is unlikely to support a comprehensive outcomes management system.

Fax servers are a variation on scannable software systems. A fax machine is in itself a scanner. The fax server functions as a remote scanner so that the central data collection center is less burdened by the transfer of paper. However, shifting burden back to the clinical sites is unlikely to improve participation. Also, fax transmission is more expensive than bulk rate mailing. The role of fax transmission for outcomes measurement systems is likely to be limited.

Patient Information Systems and Electronic Medical Records

The growth of patient information systems, including electronic medical records (EMR), scheduling, billing, and clinical laboratory systems, means that a significant amount of data is available in electronic form. Although EMRs are currently used in only a small percentage of office- and hospital-based medical practices (estimated at less than 5 percent in 1998; Amatayakul, 1998), that number is expected to grow substantially over the next five years. These systems, however, do not necessarily solve the problem, for the following reasons:

- Most EMRs are not yet integrated with scheduling, billing, or clinical systems because they have been created by different and proprietary vendors.
- The structured data collection necessary for outcomes management has not been embedded into the systems and requires customized authoring.
- There is inconsistency in data dictionaries not only between systems but within the same system at different sites. Therefore, although the potential is there, EMRs have not yet fulfilled their promise of making outcomes assessment easier.

Improvements in data replication and transformation technologies will help to integrate diverse patient information systems. The consolidation of vendors will decrease the amount of customization necessary to support the same basic data collection in different sites. Pressure from consumers to have access to authoring tools and database structures will enable medical practices to use the systems they have invested in better. If a medical practice is investing in patient information systems to improve outcomes management, outcomes expertise should be sought in the planning stages, prior to that investment. Finally, medical practices should anticipate the need to export outcomes data to larger databases for comparative purposes. These databases should work across multiple types of information platforms because any one system provider is unlikely to have an unbiased repository to provide these comparisons in a meaningful way.

Direct Data Mobile Devices

Mobile data entry systems seek to avoid duplicate data entry and paper. Typically, mobile devices use the wireless transfer of electronic patient information from the device to a central database. The purpose of these systems in the medical setting is to bring the data entry closer to the point of care and make data entry more efficient for the provider. Mobile data entry systems are then linked to the patient information system or to a dedicated database. In some cases, the transfer signals (such as in the cellular telephone ranges) can disrupt certain medical devices, so shielding is required. Hand-held devices that store and later download data or transmit data directly provide a data entry device at the point of care and therefore decrease the need for paper. These devices also provide a means to deliver outcomes management information back to the clinician at the point of care, meaning that processed information can be delivered from a central source back to the devices. The temporal relationship of outcomes management information to the point of care is an important determinant of whether such information will influence the care given. Although the potential is large, these devices are currently an extension of patient information systems/EMRs and have the same limitations.

Touch Screens

Touch-screen technologies offer a relatively simple approach to patient-based data entry in the office setting and can eliminate part of the paper trail. Touch screens can also present large-font patient-based surveys and surveys in multiple languages, facilitating the initial or follow-up health status survey (providing that the patient returns to the office or clinic or hospital). The advantages of touch-screen technologies for data entry depend on the age of the patient and the degree of infirmity.

Interactive Voice Recognition Technology

Despite a surge in the use of computers and Internet access, telephones outnumber computers in every country in the world. Interactive voice recognition software (IVR) uses voice and telephone keypad punching to transmit data over telephone lines to computers. It thus leverages the telephone as a keyboard for geographically distributed data entry.

IVR is relatively cost-efficient. Multiple telephone lines can be handled by a single computer workstation. IVR systems can generate and query databases. As such, IVR systems have been used for data entry in physician offices and by patients from home, an appealing alternative to mailing follow-up surveys or scheduling telephone calls. Until recently, IVR has been limited by the need to enter data into the telephone handset, so long surveys become extremely burdensome. However, improvement in voice recognition and the ability of such software systems to have "discrete" or continuous voice recognition allows for greater flexibility in questionnaire delivery and interactivity.

Internet

The Internet, a new and important format for outcomes measurement and management, provides significant advantages for outcomes management. It is geographically indifferent, stores data in a large central database that is accessible for day-to-day use, provides information nearly in real time, does not require significant investment by the end user in hardware or software, is scalable from tens to thousands of users, and is a platform that is being developed and widely distributed for other purposes. The Internet provides a mechanism for connectivity. It does not, however, eliminate end user issues surrounding duplication of effort.

The compelling advantage of the Internet as a system for outcomes management rests in the efficiencies of a centralized rather than a distributed model. A distributed model involves stand-alone software that is distributed to each participating site. In a centralized system, geographically distributed medical practices work simultaneously with the same database, so changes made centrally are immediately replicated throughout the network. There is no reshipping of systems to the sites. Additional studies are added quickly and efficiently. Support is less expensive because it is performed centrally. The system can differentiate one user from another, a function that facilitates comparative reporting and customized data analysis. In addition, because data are central and available for real-time analysis, outcomes feedback can be delivered to the clinician on demand, increasing the likelihood that information will arrive near the point of care to improve medical decision making. It gives even small medical practices access and participation in larger outcomes networks.

The Internet can be integrated with all of the enabling technologies, to allow flexibility in data entry, storage, analysis, and delivery. Nevertheless, there are several limiting factors in the use of the Internet for outcomes studies:

- Large studies require significant bandwidth and server space to maintain reasonable speed.
- There are peculiarities or instabilities associated with the Internet, including differences in browsers, firewalls, and the indirect path of the Internet itself, which can create significant problems and expense.
- Web databases for outcomes studies are two way, meaning that all the data are entered via the web as well as stored and retrieved. Providing a centralized two-way web database architecture that is functional, reliable, and scalable requires experience and expertise that is very different from that required for hosting one-way web databases. Many institutions and groups have already wasted significant resources exploring Internet data collection, only to find that the expertise required for web databasing is different than that offered by most vendors.

In addition to technological issues, the Internet poses several problems for outcomes and medical data in general, among them security, physician confidentiality, and patient privacy. As a public network, security and privacy issues occur at the data source, in transfer, and at the data target or repository. Security and privacy concerns start with the view screen in a medical office: what information is displayed and who can see it. Access is another security issue and is addressed through protective mechanisms including passwords and electronic signatures. Data transfer involves multiple connections via a routing process that provides an opportunity for computers not directly involved to access the data. Current software provides protection through security layers and encryption. However, secure transfer does not mean that the information that reaches the data repository is itself safe. The data repository must have its own security layer to prevent manipulation or theft. Fortunately, most of the data security issues have been addressed for commerce and for other confidential transactions; hence, the required software is readily available. Privacy and confidentiality concerns for both the patient and the physician may involve legal restrictions, which can differ from state to state and across international borders. Ensuring privacy and confidentiality requires significant forethought and planning.

Despite these limitations, the Internet provides advantages that cannot be replicated by any other data collection and reporting strategy. Actually these limitations are not unique to the Internet, but extend to all other networked databases. Coupled with the rapid assimilation of the Internet into our daily lives, improving technologies for pushing and pulling information, and the incredible pace of expanding access and bandwidth, there is no doubt that the Internet will play an increasingly significant role in the future of medical outcomes assessment.

Reference

Amatayakul, M. "The State of the Computer-Based Patient Record." *Journal of AHIMA*, 1998, *69*.

Chapter Nine

Data Management in Outcomes

Joseph T. Branca

Outcomes assessment is a data-intensive process. The real "value-adds" obtainable from outcomes measurement systems, in terms of management, improvement, benchmarking, and bringing information to the point of care, are made possible by the relatively recent technological revolution in data management. The promise, problems, and pitfalls that face outcomes data managers are those inherent in converting large databases into an entity known in the information technology industry as the data warehouse, which is a central repository of data that are in a format that can be readily mined for information. Physicians, acting as organizational decision makers in outcomes management decisions, should have some familiarity with these concepts, which have become critical to the effective implementation of outcomes measurement, management, and improvement systems.

Data management includes a number of activities, from data collection and entry through data warehousing and mining. Although a simple outcomes study may require no more than a spreadsheet, an outcomes management system typically requires a more substantial data management infrastructure. This chapter examines the key elements of data management: data collection, database technology, data warehousing, and data mining.

Data Collection or Data Capture

The process of determining the information that should populate a database is a significant part of the data management process.

A database must be comprehensive in scope and should satisfy the need for rapid dissemination of information. For a database that will be used to interact with clinicians, the danger lies in cluttering it with excess and redundant data. Excess data reduce efficiency and can slow the response time of the database. For the health care industry, the degree and scope of data collection will vary with the organization's focus.

Data collection is designed at the front end as retrospective or prospective. *Retrospective* outcomes measures capture data by looking back at specific instances in a patient's clinical history. *Prospective* measures collect data for months or years following treatment to provide ongoing data collection up to a clinical end point. Prospective outcomes information compares different physician services to determine which course of treatment is better correlated to improved patient outcomes. The process of collecting prospective outcomes data is more tedious, but the "value-add" of the results is significant.

Retrospective data capture runs the risk of becoming data dredging (the flawed, non-hypothesis-driven collection and analysis that looks for any statistical associations). For example, vendors have developed software packages to extract "outcomes" information from current standardized hospital data tracking systems for reimbursement claims. These vendors have sophisticated computer algorithms to interpret claims data, including information on length of hospital stay, codes for primary and secondary diagnoses, and mortality rates. These data are being used for purposes other than those for which they were intended, thus the term *data dredging.* Algorithms cannot improve the quality of the raw data that have been designed for claims adjudication and entered by clerks. Risk adjustment is retrospective, based on diagnostic codes, and derived health "outcomes" run the risk of being neither condition specific nor clinically meaningful.

Prospective data collection requires a data management system that is unobtrusive to clinical practice. Structured data collection can be programmed into the database to allow for validated data entry. Data are collected for an extended period of time that is clinically meaningful for the condition under evaluation. Data that specifically measure the quality of medical outcomes are collected throughout. Prospective studies typically collect data points at several intervals after the patient has left the health care setting. For example, in addition to the information gathered prior to and during any medical intervention, patients and providers may be contacted for data collection six, twelve, and even eighteen months or more after treatment. The additional information gathered before treatment and after discharge is invaluable for assessing quality clinical outcomes, because outcomes are defined by change in health status. The data are risk adjusted to account for differences between patients in both disease severity and known risk factors for disease progression. This prevents inappropriate assignment of a poor outcome to a process or provider that is actually attributable to the patient's own likelihood of disease progression or treatment failure. Collecting data for months and years instead of days or weeks after medical intervention has overwhelming benefits to the value and accuracy of information collected.

A 1994 report by the Joint Commission on Accreditation of Healthcare Organizations distinguished between intermediate outcomes, such as those collected by retrospective studies (biochemical, physiological, anatomical, and histological outcomes), and clinical outcomes, which are collected by prospective studies (reduced mortality, improved physical functioning, lessened symptoms).

Data that are planned, prospective, and collected for the purpose of a given study have great value in an outcomes database and as part of a data warehouse. Data mining tools can be employed to establish data relationships and predictions for clinical outcomes. Retrospective data can supplement prospective outcomes data, but should not be used as an alternative because they are not condition specific and may not be interpretable clinically. Retrospective data are useful for studies concerned with reimbursement claims, mortality, acute morbidity, and risk adjustment, but ultimately prospective outcomes will provide the most useful information for proving quality of care.

Object Versus Relational Databases

Collecting outcomes and administrative data is only the first step in data management. Data must be organized in databases to provide timely access to decision making. Determining how the data should be stored and represented is an important issue. Software vendors offer many different database products, which generally fall into two categories: object oriented or relational oriented. Object-oriented databases store complex data and relationships among the data elements directly in the database, such as a data element with a specific mathematical function. Relational databases map information to relational columns and rows. Relational databases continue to hold a dominant market share, but the object-oriented movement is beginning to gain user acceptance (Cattell, 1994).

Object database development was sparked because of the limitations in managing complex data, such as multimedia applications, with relational database technology. Object databases are able to store information as objects that are linked to other data elements, whereas traditional relational databases store data in rows in a table that must be linked to other relational-oriented rows and columns. In addition to traditional relational-oriented information, object-oriented technology enables built-in functions and methods to be stored.

The arrival of object databases allowed data to be represented as they appear in real-world applications, so users are not confined to the geometric limitations of a table of rows and columns. Object database advantages are seen in powerful applications of the new data types. They offer more powerful and rapid querying and decrease server loads. In addition, object technology bridges the gap between databases and the Internet. Relational databases have yet to incorporate functionality with web servers. Object technology has been readily accepted for multimedia industries, financial trading, and even health care because of its ability to handle complex data types and interact with the Internet. The movement to replace relational databases completely, however, has not occurred.

Relational databases remain the most common platform for data storage. Microsoft, Oracle, and Sybase are continually improving the functionality and power of these traditional databases. Data are normalized and stored in tables, and query functions link the tables and similar fields. For large, integrated warehouses, relational technology may be more practical. Object technology offers advantages only for specialized, complex data types and may not be suitable for legacy data.

Data Warehousing

The next step in data management is the development of active systems for using stored data to improve clinical decision making. This requires the development of a data warehouse. The technology for data warehousing is well developed in other industries. Integrated and easily accessible database management systems (DBMS) provide information regarding services that enables management to make timely decisions and improve productivity and efficiency. Health care has lagged behind other industries in the movement to build data warehouses primarily because the concept of documenting and examining the value of products and services is new to the industry.

Increasing competition due to cost pressures and managed care is forcing health care organizations to produce data that can support and prove the quality of their services. As cost and patient satisfaction begin to shape health care delivery, the industry is becoming much more business oriented. Unfortunately hospital legacy information systems, based on mainframe computers, hinder access to valuable information. Thus, there is a rapidly growing need for data warehouses, which will be vital to the survival of all types of health care organizations. Many organizations have already started to develop the infrastructure that will help reduce the costs of managing and delivering quality health care.

A simple DBMS can begin with a data repository (or database). Organizing data into a database is the first step toward converting the data into useful and valuable information. Today's databases allow enormous amounts of information to be accessible and manageable with the rapid improvements in microprocessor speeds and storage capacities of the personal computer. The repository is a passive participant and acts only as a storage facility, but the data in today's repositories are significantly more accessible and manageable than data stored in outdated legacy systems. Legacy systems are being replaced by client-server architecture that allows for greater flexibility in data transfer, analysis, and backup. Client-server applications can function in a local area network (LAN) environment that connects desktop PCs within an organization using multiple servers (see Figure 9.1). Servers are simply computers that distribute information to desktop PCs when it is needed

Figure 9.1. Local Area Network Architecture.

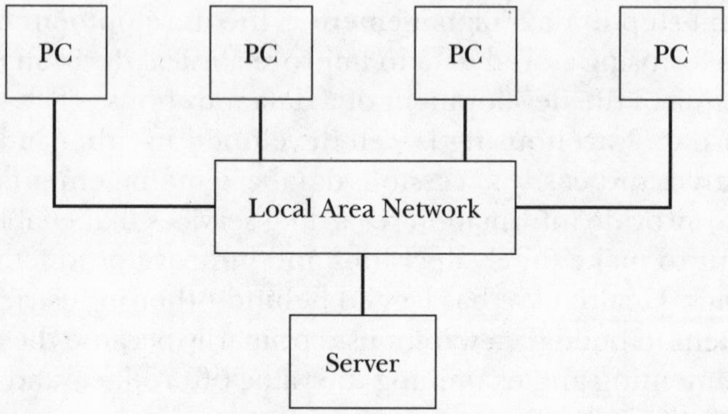

---

by an end user. This type of open architecture enables an organization to share data with multiple end users easily.

Accessing data stored on servers via a desktop PC has drastically changed the way that data are managed and analyzed and has reduced the time required to get results. In addition, even users with limited computer knowledge can rapidly produce comprehensive queries and reports using powerful, user-friendly software tools.

Unfortunately, the information stored in databases is not always accessible to an entire organization. A health care organization may have many data repositories that contain varying degrees of administrative and clinical information. A hospital may have separate surgical scheduling, laboratory, pharmacy, and clinical data systems. Maintaining patient information in electronic form is valuable to a health care organization, but as separate entities, these repositories have limited value and act as isolated islands of information.

It is an inefficient use of resources to maintain isolated data repositories. Isolated data sources are not readily accessible to end users, nor do they provide an enterprise view of an organization. Moreover, the end user has no way of knowing where specific data are stored. Instead of simply transferring data electronically through a network, hard copies must be rereviewed, a process that involves time-consuming chart reviews and redundant data entry. Manual data abstraction and entry in another system increases the likelihood of error and undermines the data quality.

To improve business and clinical decision-making processes, a health care organization must have timely access to integrated, consistent information. To achieve this, repositories must be linked and accessible to end users in many locations. Linking the sources of information by building a data warehouse can save time and money by simplifying the process of converting raw data to useful information.

Data Uses and Modeling

A data warehouse is not a single product that can be purchased. Rather, it is a system for managing multiple sources of data so that they can be collected and analyzed in the most efficient manner possible.

Development of a data warehouse requires extensive strategic planning. The planning begins with and is shaped by the information needs of the business or practice and the end users of that information. Since the financial investment can be significant, on the order of millions of dollars, the planning cannot be taken lightly and must be focused on developing a system that will best suit the needs of the organization (Ladaga, 1995). Before the architecture and technological components of the system are considered, all potential applications and objectives must be well thought out. Many data warehousing projects fail because the planners lack the necessary understanding to implement the appropriate system (Hildebrand, 1995; Lardear, 1995).

All data sources must be identified. End users must be involved in the planning process to determine the types of queries and reports that are needed. Users of a hospital's data warehouse, for instance, need readily accessible financial, clinical, and outcomes data to make quick and informed decisions about a patient's health or to modify and improve procedures and policies.

Planning and understanding all of the uses of a data warehouse can be extremely difficult for a health care organization. Identifying and prioritizing business objectives are difficult because the industry's direction is unclear. Industry restructuring will affect many organizations. Consolidation can quickly change the long- and short-term objectives of a health care organization. The formation of geographically distributed physician networks increases the complexity of a data warehousing project. Ultimately sharing of data across geographic barriers will be accomplished with wide area networks and the use of the Internet. Web integration, however, adds a new dimension to data warehousing requirements.

It is difficult enough to clean (or align data elements and definitions) and generate the consistency that will be essential to a properly functioning warehouse with data coming from multiple sources at one location. When data enter a warehouse from multiple locations, the complexity multiplies. Fortunately, an organization attempting to function as a single unit across its many locations can obtain substantial rewards from a well-designed data warehouse. Creating a data warehouse that can be accessed by users at multiple locations enables an organization to provide consistent, quality health care through a truly integrated delivery system.

Data modeling, or the process of choosing the data elements and definitions, is a key issue. For a data warehouse to achieve its full potential, the data elements must be consistent. A protocol must be established for data entry and cleansing to meet the standards of the data model. For health care organizations, this process requires that health care providers be involved in any data warehousing project. It is important that the data model make sense to those who provide the care and those charged with the data entry responsibility. Ideally the physician would enter data at the time of treatment to ensure data integrity. Currently the best alternative is to develop a straightforward and consistent model for coding and entering data. The difficulty lies in the lack of standardization in coding systems across the health care industry.

Multiple coding systems for coding procedures, discharge diagnoses, clinical data, and prescriptions are used within and between health care organizations. A data warehouse must be able to reconcile differences in data elements to maximize the value of the information it produces. For instance, the sex of a patient may be coded as "1" or "2" in one database but as "m" or "f" in another database. Creating and agreeing on a comprehensive, user-friendly data model and cleansing all data coming into a data warehouse to meet that model is a difficult but essential task.

Architectural Planning

After the data model and objectives for a data warehouse have been thought out, architectural planning begins. A warehouse includes both software and hardware components on a platform that is scalable to allow for flexibility and growth as user demand increases. Hardware platforms must be carefully chosen. Instead, they often are chosen based on the servers and legacy systems that are currently in place.

Multiple sources feed data into a warehouse architecture, where they are processed and made accessible to many different end users. Software applications for both the servers and PCs are chosen based on usage requirements and system demands for transportation and transformation of the data. Generally the movement and manipulation of data through a warehouse follows a pattern involving these essential functions:

1. Specific data elements are extracted from their sources.
2. Data elements are cleansed to reconcile differences and generate a consistent data model.
3. Cleansed data elements are consolidated and summarized.
4. Data are transported from various sources to populate the data warehouse.
5. Querying and data mining tools are used to examine data for valuable information.

With each component performing integral functions, choosing warehouse management tools that are compatible across the different hardware platforms demands an elaborate architectural plan. An additional concern is the incorporation of valuable data from legacy systems, such as a mainframe computer. Health care legacy systems provide challenges for determining which platforms will be used for the warehouse so that data existing in legacy systems can be loaded into the new warehouse architecture. LAN-based client-server applications may provide a flexible link enabling access to a mainframe from a PC. In this case the legacy data become an integral part of the LAN environment. Alternatively, the mainframe could be converted to a server that is accessed by the LAN-based client-server architecture. Either possibility poses significant challenges before data elements can be cleansed and transported from their original sources to the data warehouse.

Many health care–specific tools have been introduced as decision support applications for a data warehouse. Data warehousing in health care, however, is a new concept, so there has been no single vendor that can offer a complete solution for a health care organization's needs. Choosing the right combination of software tools and hardware can be somewhat of a gamble. Flexibility and scalability are necessary attributes in warehouse architecture to meet new demands on the warehouse.

In addition to constructing the warehouse, there are significant maintenance issues to be addressed. A data warehouse is not a stagnant storage facility. Security, recovery, and backup procedures are essential to the viability of the system. Staff must be trained to manage the system, and end users must be trained to use the system effectively. The data warehouse is most efficient if the end users of its information are decision makers in the organization who can quickly act on newly discovered information. But training issues increase costs on systems that already come with exorbitant price tags.

The full benefits of a data warehouse are not immediately realized. Lengthy development and maintenance issues act as deterrents to leaping into data warehouse development (Redding, 1995). Is the data warehouse worth the investment? Industry estimates place the return on investment at 400 percent for data warehouses that are planned and used properly (Depriest, 1997). Successful data warehouses are integral to decision-making processes and can ultimately shape the way an organization is run.

Data Elements

There are several key differences between source data and the data that enter a warehouse (McDonald, Overhage, Dexter, Takesue, and Dwyer, 1997):

- Data existing on PCs are known as *operational data;* data entering a warehouse are *analytical data.*
- Operational data are updated and recent; analytical data are nonvolatile, read-only, and may be several years old.
- The transition from the operational environment to the data warehouse cleanses the data; it also separates application-oriented data and stores them as subject-oriented data. In other words, data on a PC are stored in the manner in which they were entered, meaning associated with the application. This

is operationally more efficient. However, in the data warehouse, the emphasis is on subject categorization, because this makes analysis more efficient.

- Operational data are critical to the daily functions of an organization. Subject-oriented, analytical data are less volatile, and crucial for making strategic decisions.
- There is very little overlap between the data contained in a warehouse and those found in the operational environment. The warehouse environment also contains stores of summary data that never existed in the operational environment.

A data warehouse acts to free PC operating systems of excessive stores of data that can interfere with the performance of the systems. Analytical data are effectively separated from constantly changing operational data. In many legacy data storage systems, storage constraints forced excess mainframe analytical data to be stored elsewhere. Unfortunately the result was that complex queries and multidimensional analyses could not be performed in a reasonable amount of time. Modern data warehouses free operating systems of large data stores, yet make the data readily available for analysis and reports.

Operational and analytical data differ in structure and functionality. Operational data are tactical in nature and are needed to run day-to-day activities of a business. Analytic data are used for strategic decision making. Operational, or "raw," data, such as those found in a pharmacy system, are updated daily with each prescription that is written and dispensed. These "operational" databases contain vast amounts of information, some of it irrelevant to decision-making processes. Converting operational data to analytical data stored in the warehouse requires data cleansing and transformation. The resulting analytical data can be accurately used to identify data relationships and trends much more rapidly than is possible with legacy systems.

Data warehouse software tools extract data from operational systems and cleanse and reconcile the elements to conform to the data model set forth in the warehouse design. The cleansing function is responsible for coding for missing information and checking the integrity of the data elements. Reconciliation transforms the data into standardized elements, eliminating data discrepancies due to differences in their source applications or coding variations. In health care organizations, for example, CPT (current procedural terminology) codes and ICD-9 (the International Classification of Diseases, ninth revision) codes must be recognized and reconciled for consistency.

Generating consistency in the data elements is essential for a manageable warehouse. The warehouse tools can recognize data relationships and properly aggregate the information. Data extracted from multiple sources can then be summarized to generate data describing the data, known as *metadata*.

Unification of large amounts of data in a warehouse poses problems for the end user interested only in generating specific reports. The data must be organized in a manner that enables rapid retrieval and efficiency. In addition to the important analytical data, a warehouse stores metadata. Metadata act as a map or table of contents for all of the data stored in the warehouse and have several important functions, including the following (Dilly, 1995):

- Providing information as to where different types of data are stored
- Identifying the different components of the warehouse and defining which areas of the warehouse are accessible to specific end users
- Specifying where data came from originally
- Providing time estimates for end user query requests

Data warehouse servers can be programmed to automate reports that end users demand on a regular basis. Once the data elements are reconciled, aggregated, and summarized, predetermined algorithms can produce standardized reports. Reports on patient outcomes, dispensed prescriptions, and operational costs, for example, can be automatically produced on a regular basis. These prototyping, querying, and reporting tools increase an organization's efficiency and allow more time for discovering complex data relationships for timely and competitive decisions.

Data Mining

A data warehouse is of little use if no significant relationships or patterns can be discovered in the data. Once the data elements are collected, cleaned, reconciled, and transported, queries and reports can be generated on which analysis can be performed. The process of analyzing, or "drilling the data down," in search of statistical relationships is known as *data mining*.

The development of analytical software tools for data mining is growing rapidly to meet the demands of businesses seeking to discover meaningful trends in their customer data. In theory, data mining will unveil data relationships that prove to be extremely valuable to an organization. Identifying patterns and trends in data can help increase revenues, operating efficiency, and customer satisfaction. Data mining is being used for many clinical applications to help predict patient outcomes.

Mining tools can automate the analysis process and present results that the end user can interpret. The end user is responsible for determining which relationships provide information that can benefit the organization. The scope of applications covered by the market for data mining tools is enormous. Many different classes of software tools exist—for example:

- Data visualization tools, which present the user with several different perspectives of data in user-friendly graphical displays
- Knowledge discovery tools, which help end users establish relationships among the data elements
- Neural networks, a class of software tools with the ability to learn from typical trends within a database

A rapidly growing area of data mining is the neural network class of software tools. Neural networks consist of mathematical algorithms that are designed to simulate neural pathways artificially in the human body. Using nonlinear mathematics, this software can effectively build data models that can be used for predicting data relationships and discovering solutions for optimal performance. In business these algorithms are effective predictors of sales and financial forecasting.

Recently these powerful neural network software tools have been applied to medical data for predicting outcomes. Applications include predicting the outcomes for radiation therapy, stroke, breast cancer, hip replacement, kidney transplantation, and myocardial infarction, to name a few (Burke, 1994; Ebell, 1993). Neural networks can replace or be used in addition to traditional logistic regression models for analysis. Having the ability to learn from trends in data, neural networks become powerful predictors of complex relationships. For medical data, neural networks can learn typical outcomes of medical interventions and aid in diagnosing particular diseases. The results can be particularly useful to physicians in deciding if medical intervention will be beneficial to a patient.

There are vast applications for data mining tools in the health care industry. HMOs use data mining to analyze trends of data describing their geographically distributed providers. Pharmaceutical companies use data mining tools to generate information that will aid in the lengthy Food and Drug Administration drug approval process and sales and marketing forecasts. Hospitals can analyze outcomes data to help benchmark procedures and reduce costs in the capitated managed care environment. Most health care organizations, however, do not use data mining tools to take advantage of their enormous data stores, which could be used to predict costs, outcomes, or length of stay.

The power in data mining is realized in its ability to generate valuable information from previously unused data elements and relationships. The danger of data mining lies in false associations and bias. Sophisticated data mining tools can discover numerous data relationships, but determining which relationships are valid and valuable is difficult. Aimless sifting through the vast amounts of information contained in a data warehouse is referred to as data dredging. Dredging through the data is time-consuming and may generate biased conclusions based on random associations. Data mining is criticized because many of the relationships it unearths are considered too random.

The data mining process should be able to detect relationships in a data warehouse that can be extremely valuable to an organization. Discovering new trends in data logically results in further data collection and analysis to support these discoveries. Thus, acting on potentially false associations is time-consuming and costly. The danger exists in the tendency to rely on a data mining tool for answers. Can the fate of a patient's course of treatment be left to a software tool? In health care especially, there is a burden of examining the results for validity.

To avoid false associations and bias in data mining, the process must be hypothesis driven. The complexities of data mining tools can create problems for an inexperienced user if allowed to run unchecked. If the end user is familiar with the data and has a clearly stated hypothesis in mind, determining which relationships are valid and which are random is simplified. Often, checking results for statistical validity is all that is required to avoid acting on false data relationships.

In the end, the information that data mining produces will be only as good as the quality of data that it came from. The costs of building a data warehouse are significant enough without the added data dredging costs. Sound data collection and data mining protocols are needed to tap into the full scope of benefits that a data warehouse can provide.

Data Repository, Data Mart, or Data Warehouse?

Some organizations have taken a less costly approach to developing DBMS by implementing only key components or scaled-down versions of a data warehouse. For instance, clinical data repositories (CDRs) are gaining favor in the health care industry. Their value lies in the aggregation of clinical data, which are often difficult and expensive to capture. CDRs differ from data warehouses in their failure to integrate other data types, such as the important administrative data. Use of the CDR for process improvement is therefore limited in scope. Building or buying a CDR without integration into a full data warehouse scheme limits access to the full spectrum of information that is required to achieve business objectives. This is not to say that a CDR is not a valuable tool for a health care organization. CDRs store data about clinical events that can help professionals make timely decisions about appropriate care, but CDRs do not necessarily provide the flexibility for competitive decision making that is available in a data warehouse. In addition, the CDR may be just as costly. Like a data warehouse, its content must be managed and monitored. A concern with a CDR is that the organization is buying a managed database rather than building a fully functional data warehouse.

A data mart is essentially the same as a CDR. Data marts are subsets of operational data that are analyzed by specific end users, such as a department within an organization. The problem with developing data marts before a data warehouse is built is that isolated stores of information are created. Although the subsets of data may be beneficial to the particular department, uniformity and consistency problems are generated. Creating data marts is attractive to organizations as a cheaper and quicker alternative to a complete data warehouse, but building data marts and later trying to expand to a data warehouse may create architectural integration problems. Successful data warehouses are well-thought-out projects that strive to identify all potential uses before the building begins. A data mart may be a quick and easy solution, but it is a shortsighted vision of how the data can benefit the organization (Ferranti, 1998).

Several vendors claim to offer advantages over the traditional CDR in the form of newer, more comprehensive CDRs. These systems involve a distributed database system with a centralized active database that distributes all active patient information to smaller databases at care facilities (Healthvision, 1998). The system uses existing operational or legacy systems to generate a repository that includes orders, results, history, profiles of care, expected outcomes, clinical pathways, and protocols. Once the patient record becomes inactive, it is stored in a data repository, where it can be accessed for analysis. The systems are scalable and offer clinicians the benefit of quick access to clinical data. Although the new generation of CDRs offer many of the benefits desired from a data warehouse, they are not complete warehousing solutions.

A health care organization must be careful to plan the uses of its data warehouse before choosing an architecture. Some vendors may be able to provide flexible and scalable components for a data warehouse, but no vendor should be relied on to determine the appropriate system for data management. Repositories and data marts are simply components of a data warehouse providing short-term solutions.

The Future of Data Warehousing

Efficient management of the vast amounts of information that an organization must process is essential to the vitality of any provider of services or products. In the health care industry, organizations increasingly are required to make information available to consumers, purchasers, and government regulatory bodies. Rising life expectancies due to technological advances in health care and other factors have often made care too expensive for the recipients of that care. Managed care has stepped in to control costs, but reducing costs while maintaining quality is difficult. Timely information is essential to compete with other organizations offering similar quality of care.

Health care has traditionally lagged behind the business world in information technology but can no longer afford to continue to do so. To compete in an increasingly competitive environment, providers and purchasers alike must become leaders in applications of data management. Their organizations will reap the benefits of increased revenues and lower costs, but patients will be the real winners as health care delivery and quality improve.

As the Internet and multimedia applications change the way information is transmitted and viewed, both the volume and complexity of the data will increase. Most health care information systems cannot handle yesterday's data, let alone today's and tomorrow's. Organizations cannot settle for recent improvements, but rather must lay the framework for the systems of the future.

Additional issues, such as patient confidentiality, have hindered health care's implementation of accessible information through data warehouse solutions. The Internet has sparked the most criticism despite the apparent security of encrypted data transfer. Fear of compromised patient confidentiality has also delayed the implementation of electronic patient records. Electronic medical records would vastly improve a physician's ability to access patient data for diagnostic and treatment purposes. Integrating electronic patient records with data warehouses will allow physicians to access patient records from just about anywhere. This capability will revolutionize health care delivery.

The future of data warehousing has powerful capabilities for generating valuable information. Using technological advances to increase revenues and quality may be limited only by the imaginative applications for technology. Health care organizations will find that data warehousing benefits are only as good as the initiative of the organization and its will to take advantage of that initiative.

References

Burke, H. B. "Artificial Neural Networks for Cancer Research: Outcome Prediction." *Seminars in Surgery and Oncology*, 1994, *10*, 73–79.

Cattell, R.G.G. "The DBMS Wars." [http://www.computerworld.com/home/print9497.nsf/all/slcattfin]. Feb. 1994.

Depriest, T. "Are You Prepped for a Data Warehouse?" [http://www.computerworld.com/home/print9497.nsf/all/sl9706nc-3]. Jun. 1, 1997.

Dilly, R. "Data Mining: An Introduction." [http://www-pcc.qub.ac.uk/tec/courses/datamining/stu_notes/dm_book_2.html]. Dec. 1995.

Ebell, M. H. "Artificial Neural Networks for Predicting Failure to Survive Following In-Hospital Cardiopulmonary Resuscitation." *Journal of Family Practice,* 1993, *36,* 297–303.

Ferranti, M. "Data Warehouse World: The Warehouse Vs. Mart Debate." [http://www.computerworld.com/85256...f0745852564ec00773a0b?OpenDocument]. June 1998.

Healthvision Corporation. "The CareVision (Clinical Data Repository." [http://www.healthvision.com/marketing/prod-cdr.htm]. June 1998.

Hildebrand, C. "Form Follows Function." *CIO,* 1995, *9*(3), 41–52.

Ladaga, J. "Let Business Goals Drive Your Data Warehouse Effort." *Health Management Technology,* 1995, *16*(11), 26–28.

Lardear, J. "Data Warehouse Hype May Outrun Results." *Midrange Systems,* 1995, *8*(15), 3, 8.

McDonald, C. J., Overhage, J. M., Dexter, P., Takesve, B. Y., and Dwyer, D. M. "A Framework for Capturing Clinical Data Sets from Computerized Sources." *Annals of Internal Medicine,* 1997, *127,* 675–682.

Redding, A. "Warehouse Wake-Up Call." *Info World,* 1995, *17*(47), 1, 57.

Part Three

Profiting from Quality: Outcomes Strategies for Medical Practice

Richard E. Gliklich

In this part, the authors explore a number of ways to *profit from quality,* from the perspectives of individual caregivers and patients to those of organizations and society. Chapter Ten outlines a series of short-term and long-term incentives that may motivate physicians to participate in outcomes management. It also describes a series of incremental strategies toward adopting an outcomes management philosophy for a practice or organization.

In Chapter Eleven, concrete steps toward implementing an outcomes initiative in a medical practice are explained. In Chapter Twelve, it is argued that the capacity to measure health and improve care is most effective at the organizational level. The organizations described may be any grouping of physicians or practices—economic, academic, or virtual. A description of organizational behavior, motivation, and planning is presented to help provide the skill set necessary to implement outcomes strategies. But if outcomes management is to be successful, data must influence change. Chapter Thirteen cites evidence on how to maximize the effectiveness of data in improving care. Turning to the practical impact of adopting an outcomes management strategy, in Chapter Fourteen an expert on health care markets focuses on immediate organizational gains from outcomes and quality measurement. Finally, Chapter Fifteen presents the personal experience and success of a medical practitioner implementing an outcomes management program.

Chapter Ten

Outcomes Incentives and Strategies for Medical Practice

Richard E. Gliklich

Physicians and medical organizations should implement outcomes and quality measurement in daily practice for a number of reasons. In the long term, arming physicians with the ability to monitor quality may provide the collective capacity to thwart economic imperatives from changing what Uwe Reinhardt and May Tsung-mei Cheng describe in Chapter One as the quality of life of health care providers as well as that of their patients. In the short term there are already significant benefits to be considered. This chapter examines ways in which medical practices may benefit from outcomes measurement and presents a number of strategies that can be considered for applying outcomes management principles to medical practice. Some of these strategies are applicable for all medical practices, while others are practical for only larger, integrated organizations.

Incentives for Participating in Quality Measurement and Improvement

Although patients benefit from a health care system, organization, or individual practice that is improved in terms of quality, it is less clear to what extent anyone is willing to pay for it. Therefore, in an era of decreasing reimbursements and higher patient volumes, introducing any program into a medical practice that requires additional work by overworked staff must provide a short-term benefit as well as longer-term gain. Physicians and health care organizations best respond to incentives to participate in quality measurement and improvement.

In the short term, there are several ways that medical practices may directly or indirectly profit from outcomes measurement.

- Data for defense. Physicians are currently being measured and profiled by health insurers and others, and this information is being used in some regions for contracting decisions. In the future, performance data may be used to determine relative reimbursement rates as well. A medical practice that is thinking about adopting an outcomes management strategy should consider that proving quality of care may become as important to the bottom line as proving that the care has been provided.

- Data for marketing. For better or for worse, data on quality and outcomes are being used increasingly for marketing purposes (see Chapters Fourteen and Fifteen).

- Data for assuming risk. Most outcomes studies can be crafted to examine costs as well as quality and performance issues. For a medical practice that is assuming risk contracts, data are critical to management and contracting. Outcomes measurement systems provide information on case mix and can be integrated with cost accounting strategies.

- Data for practice management. In addition to quality improvement, outcomes measurement provides data useful for practice management. Practice success is a function of both the quality of the product and the efficiencies of the management. Outcomes data support the efficiencies of management because they enable a practice to manage with data.

- Sharing data. There is a growing demand for information on quality. Outcomes data collected by medical practices create value for multiple groups. Outcomes data collection creates opportunities to develop health care information partners or groups that can mutually benefit from the same data. Sharing data can offset the costs of data collection for medical practices or provide additional revenue to those practices.

In the long term, medical practices will benefit from outcomes measurement by using measurement to improve medical practice and by reestablishing the physician's role as conveyor of health quality information and guardian of health care quality.

Choosing Strategies

The ultimate value of outcomes measurement lies in its capacity to improve care. Each practice or organization may choose from several potential strategies for implementing outcomes measurement to meet regulatory or competitive needs or to use in decision support. A practice or organization that is choosing a strategy should ask itself these questions:

- Are there demands on the organization or practice to produce outcomes information for regulatory compliance?
- Is there a competitive need to produce either patient satisfaction data or true outcomes information to secure contracts or for marketing purposes?
- Is there organizational support for collecting outcomes data? What is the financial commitment to collecting outcomes data? What is the physicians' level of interest in and commitment to collecting data? What is the staff's level of interest in and commitment to collecting data?
- What is the level of organizational understanding of outcomes measurement and its applications?
- What are the organization's strategic goals for the effort?

There are six possible strategies to choose from. The outcomes strategies presented here begin with a focus on meeting external pressures for comparative information and competitive needs and progress to a focus on internal reengineering that more significantly affects the production of quality health care for the practice or the organization.

Do Nothing

The "do nothing" strategy is a cost-effective option. It argues that the demands for outcomes information are ill defined, and the up-front costs of pursuing a sophisticated outcomes management or improvement system are not a sound investment.

Measure Patient Satisfaction

Patient satisfaction is the "customer service" component of health care delivery. There are compelling reasons in the health care marketplace to measure and improve patient satisfaction. Since satisfaction is more closely correlated to professional services and facilities than to disease, patient satisfaction data has immediate utility without requiring complex analyses. It also does not require clinician or medical record input into the data set. In addition, many health plans require participating providers to provide some sort of satisfaction data.

Patient satisfaction measurement is appealing. Well-constructed satisfaction measures that are given at regular intervals in medical practice settings can yield significant information regarding customer-related issues. Since satisfaction can be correlated closely with services, there is an opportunity to use satisfaction information to continuously improve the facility and the professional interactions. Comparative data from other practitioners and facilities are also useful in understanding service issues. Longitudinal data collection provides an opportunity to understand the impact of service interventions on patient satisfaction. For example, the introduction of a valet parking service or a change in office scheduling patterns can be readily assessed for the impact on patient satisfaction if appropriate measures and methodologies for data collection and analysis are used.

Measure Clinical Processes

Clinical pathways and guidelines are evidence-based summaries of best practices. Although typically abstracted from other health systems or untested in terms of quality measurement, these process support tools can be tracked. Understanding compliance and variation from clinical pathways is a useful mechanism for process improvement and thereby quality improvement. In many cases and for many conditions, measurement of true health outcomes is not practical or even possible, and measurement of clinical processes provides the best approach to measuring quality.

Measure Health Outcomes

The collection of general health data is useful and is an important addition to patient satisfaction. It yields an estimate of the relative burden of disease across the population being seen in a facility or practice versus normative standards or other facilities or practices. It provides baseline health status measurements that can be followed along with treatment or interventions over time.

Condition-specific measurement systems include more disease-specific information, are generally more sensitive to clinical change with therapy, and together with general health measures provide an overall picture of the patient and the illness.

Create Outcomes Management Systems

Outcomes management systems require the use of general and condition-specific measures, appropriate staging, and feedback to stimulate change. Outcomes management systems are therefore condition or intervention specific. What differentiates outcomes management systems from measurement systems alone is the feedback loop. Information must be returned to the providers so that they can learn from it and act on it. Outcomes management systems require an investment in infrastructure for data collection and reporting that can range from limited to extensive.

Create Outcomes Improvement Systems

Outcomes improvement systems are a variation on outcomes management systems that use more rigorous approaches to quantifying processes and analyzing the relationship between processes and outcomes. Detailing processes for a condition may include monitoring clinical pathways for variance, detailing surgical procedures, and closely documenting variations among physicians. Outcomes improvement systems require measurement systems with high levels of responsiveness in order to determine significant differences between processes or variations. Statistical techniques to generate composite outcome indexes are one approach to achieving highly responsive measures that can be used for outcome improvement systems.

Data feedback plays the critical role in outcomes improve-ment systems. Clinicians and administrators are presented with statistical evidence that describes both processes and variations and the predictive value of each for both outcomes and cost. This can have a profound impact on altering clinician behavior and for understanding cost-quality trade-offs. Importantly, outcomes improvement systems make use of existing variations in the system to cause evolutionary change by selecting for variations that lead to better outcomes.

Six Sigma Health Care Quality

An even more active model of outcomes improvement, borrowed from industrial examples, we have termed six sigma health care quality. The term *six sigma quality* refers to the distribution about the mean of a process or procedure. In manufacturing, average processes function at about three sigma level, or 66,807 defects per million opportunities. A six sigma level translates to fewer than 3.4 defects per million opportunities.[1] Although the level of quality sought for jet engines may not be translatable to gall bladder surgery, the concept of six sigma as an approach to quality improvement can be applied in health care as an extension of the concepts of outcomes improvement systems.

The challenge is to improve health care further. Turning to the normal distribution, there is some minimal standard level that a particular health care organization will find tolerable. Anything below that level will be considered unacceptable in terms of health result or cost, or both. If best practice has been achieved as defined by the mean of the health measurement against a standard, then the goal of the organization shifts to narrow the distribution around the mean so that a larger portion of the distribution is above the minimal tolerance level. Therefore, the focus of reengineering shifts toward narrowing the lower tail of the distribution through care process redesign, incorporating change earlier in the process. The earlier the change is made, the lower the cost will be. As com-plex models are developed based on collected outcomes data, analy-sis will provide a means to predict for best process in design.

In six sigma health care quality, the following principles are followed:

- All aspects of care are rigorously catalogued through best practices, guidelines, clinical pathways, process flow charts, and so on.
- An emphasis is placed on using outcomes measurement systems that provide indexes that can be studied using the six sigma methodology.
- Best-practice standards are developed for the condition and the intervention. Rather than implying an unreachable quality level, this means that the standard level is determined and a decision is made on how to push that quality to the next level.
- All available data are used to assist teams that will use the information to transform processes at the front end.

As in six sigma industrial models, tribal knowledge is repudiated in favor of the data. The goal is to achieve a culture of quality improvement based on process quantification, outcomes measurement, and continual use of data. This approach requires a tremendous investment in training and infrastructure and a highly sophisticated approach to outcomes measurement systems.

Note

1. Six sigma is a concept of quality improvement used in manufacturing. For example, if one is making pipes and the ideal diameter of the pipe is 4 cm, then there will be a normal distribution of what is actually produced around 4 cm. Some pipes will be 4.1 cm and some may be 3.9 cm. At some point, the pipe diameter becomes unacceptable for use in the manufacturing process and is considered a defect. If 3.8 cm and 4.2 cm are the tolerance limits for the system, then the goal of the six sigma process is to generate a product distribution that yields only 3.4 pipes out of every 1 million that are either greater than 4.2 cm or less than 3.8 cm. From a statistical point of view, the normal distribution is narrowed (Pryzdek, 1996). If one were to apply a single outcomes measurement to the x-axis for condition z, a normal distribution is likely to occur. The mean performance of the organization is at a particular level. As one employs best practices, eventually that level becomes optimized for that particular condition.

Reference
Pryzdek, T. *The Complete Guide to CQE.* Tucson: Quality Publishing, 1996.

Chapter Eleven

Implementing Outcomes Management in Medical Practice

Megan Morgan

Despite the growing interest in outcomes, relatively few organizations have become involved in developing outcomes initiatives to improve quality and cost-effectiveness. The reasons cited for this lack of involvement vary; however, moving from the concept to its implementation is clearly a challenge.

Measurement and Improvement

There are four outcomes of any treatment intervention: clinical, functional status/quality of life, patient satisfaction, and cost. The improvement of any, or all, requires measurement. The important connection between measurement and improvement is an essential concept to bear in mind when developing an outcomes initiative. The following questions need to be asked during the initial stages of development:

- What goals are we trying to achieve by collecting outcomes data (for example, improvement of patient satisfaction, reduction of postoperative infection rates, increase in functional status, reduction of cost)?
- How will the data be collected (for example, from the patient, the physician, using claims-based data)?

- What changes within our organization need to be made to achieve our goals?
- How will we able to measure the change?
- How will we use the data collected?

The answers to these questions create a framework to identify participants (both physician and staff) to be included during the planning phase of the new initiative. In addition, a sense of the additional resources required, such as support in data collection, management and analysis, assistance in the selection or development of measures, and consultation in process improvement, will emerge.

General Principles

The initial phases of development may appear impossibly complex. One group (Nelson, Spaline, Batalden, and Plume, 1998, pp. 460–466) has recommended the following principles:

- Seek useful, not perfect, measures. Keep in mind what you are trying to measure and why. Whenever possible, use existing instruments rather than developing new measures. Use a small data set rather than collecting too many data. Keep the limitations of your resources, time, and practice environment in mind when developing the preliminary data set.
- Blend process, outcome, and cost measures. In a competitive health care environment, comparing value with cost is a prerequisite. Medical care involves an interactive system that has a number of stakeholders (the patient, family, employer, payer, and clinician), all with different interests. Including a mix of measures allows an evaluation of clinical outcome, patient-reported outcomes, and the cost of treatment.
- Think broadly, but start small. Implementing an outcomes initiative requires focus and simplicity. If your plan for implementation is too complex, it will not be followed, and your attempts to collect data will fail. Start small, and build on your successes.
- Carefully define what you are trying to measure. For example, if you are measuring the impact of conservative treatment for lower back pain, the patient might be asked, several weeks into treatment, "Are you still bothered by pain in your back?

Please answer yes or no." By defining the measures carefully, you create an efficient method for systematically measuring the key variable.

• Integrate outcomes measurement into your daily practice. The success of any office-based outcome initiative rests in part on the integration of data collection into daily practice. For example, if a nurse routinely follows up by telephone with a patient seven days after a procedure, standard questions to collect certain outcome data from the patient can be incorporated into that routine telephone call. If you are attempting to collect patient satisfaction data from patients before they leave the office, the appointment desk can remind patients to complete the survey they received on arrival at the office and drop it in a conveniently located box prior to leaving the office. Finding ways to integrate outcomes measurement into an already established routine will help enroll staff in the process of implementation.

• Develop a team. Do not attempt to implement a broad outcomes initiative by yourself. Create a team of interested clinicians and staff to share the workload. The team approach will also yield valuable input regarding the mechanics of implementation. The more members of your staff you can enroll in the process, the more successful your efforts will be.

Organizational Issues in Implementation

A number of organizational issues come into play during the development of an outcomes initiative. Although these are dealt with in more detail in subsequent chapters, following is a brief overview of pertinent issues.

• Commitment of the leadership is essential. Regardless of the size of your organization, the leadership must be strongly committed to the development and implementation of the outcomes initiative. A failure to obtain commitment will doom any initiative before it begins. If the leadership is not yet in agreement, spend the necessary time and energy to educate them, and achieve consensus before beginning development.

• Involve physicians and staff. Another key factor for success is the involvement of physicians early in the process. Efforts should be made to make physician time available by providing additional support to both the participating physicians and their colleagues left to cover clinical responsibilities. Reimbursement should positively reflect their involvement (Blumenthal and Edwards, 1995). Equally important is the involvement by nonphysician staff (both clinical and nonclinical) during all phases of planning and development. Without staff support, any data collected will be at best incomplete, and in reality, more likely not collected. In addition, nonphysician staff play a key role during implementation. Eliciting their input and suggestions during the planning stage will prevent numerous problems during implementation.

• Avoid jargon and technical terms. The design of an outcomes initiative and its use in process improvement borrows from the theories developed within the Total Quality Management (TQM) philosophy, initially an industrial model. Health care providers have been highly resistant to TQM and slow to embrace its potential application in medicine. Therefore, avoid using the jargon and technical terms associated with TQM. Emphasize the data-driven nature and scientific foundation of the process (Blumenthal and Edwards, 1995). The results will speak for themselves once data collection and analysis begin.

• Educate, educate, educate. The development and implementation of any outcomes initiative, regardless of complexity, requires knowledge and skills that the majority of physicians and their staff have not already acquired. Education and training should start simultaneously with the decision to begin planning an outcomes initiative. Developing the requisite skills is a process that takes time. Waiting until time for data collection is too long and will result in a significant delay in collecting meaningful data.

Benefits of Outcomes Initiatives

It is helpful to review examples of outcomes initiatives that were beneficial to participants. Following are three vignettes that show the utility of outcomes initiatives in a variety of settings and illustrate that they can indeed be successfully implemented. The second and third were shared by clients who have successfully used outcomes data to benefit their practice.

A moderate-size, private practice cardiac surgery group in the Midwest participated in the Society of Thoracic Surgery's database program. Using the data within the program, the practice presented a formal preferred provider organization proposal to two major industries in their community. The group profiled outcomes for all of its patients from the previous three years and prepared a separate section relating to patients employed by these two large corporations. The practice's ability to categorize the patients prospectively by risk levels convinced the companies of the practice's attention to detail and analysis of outcomes. As a result, the practice and the two companies entered into a contract that resulted in an additional 148 patient referrals from these businesses during the first year [Clark, 1995].

A gastroenterology group practiced in a southern metropolitan area saturated with other gastroenterology groups. Managed care began to penetrate the area and seek providers. This practice group had collected outcomes data, including length of stay, quality of life, patient satisfaction, and cost data, for the previous two years. Using these data, the practice successfully negotiated an exclusive provider contract with the largest managed care provider. The exclusive relationship resulted in an additional two hundred patient referrals during the first year and helped the practice create a dominant presence in a highly competitive marketplace.

A group of urologists practicing in the Los Angeles area was offered a capitated contract from a managed care organization they had been involved with for a number of years. Patients covered under this plan represented a large percentage of total patients that the practice treated. Although the capitated contract seemed economically attractive, a review of outcomes data collected over the previous twenty-four months by the practice revealed that accepting the capitated contract as offered would result in a substantial loss of income. Using the data, the group was able to negotiate a more reasonable capitated contract that maintained patient referrals at a higher level of profitability.

In these examples, the collection of data also led to improved processes improvement, increased efficiencies, and improved patient satisfaction.

A broader initiative, representative of one of the most successful applications of analyzing and feedback outcomes data to achieve health care quality improvement, follows.

In 1987, with the participation of all cardiothoracic surgeons in the region, investigators from the Northern New England Cardiovascular Disease Study Group (NNECDSG) initiated an outcomes registry of coronary artery bypass graft (CABG) surgeries performed in Maine, New Hampshire, and Vermont. By early 1990, examination of these outcomes data demonstrated that differences in the mortality rates across institutions in northern New England were not largely a consequence of differences in case mix but represented actual differences in unknown aspects of patient care.

In 1990, as a further refinement of outcomes data analysis, the NNECDSG developed a method to code the primary cause of death among CABG patients. Subsequently a series of interventions (including continuous quality improvement training, benchmarking visits, specific data feedback, and discussion) were applied in an attempt to reduce the mortality rate associated with CABG surgery. The result over a three-year period was a 24 percent postintervention reduction in the rate of thirty-day CABG-associated mortality in northern New England [O'Connor and others, 1996].

Conclusion

Establishing the beginning phases of development for a broad-based outcomes initiative is a complex endeavor. However, success is possible if careful planning takes place. Patience, persistence, and adeptly facilitating the change process will help create the momentum necessary.

References
Al-Assaf, A. F., and Schmele, J. *The Textbook of Total Quality in Healthcare.* Boca Raton, Fla.: St. Lucie Press, 1997.
Blumenthal, D., and Edwards, J. "Involving Physicians in Total Quality Management: Results of a Study." In D. Blumenthal and A. Scheck (eds.), *Improving Clinical Practice: Total Quality Management and the Physician.* San Francisco: Jossey-Bass, 1995.
Clark, R. "The STS Cardiac Surgery National Database: An Update." *Annals of Thoracic Surgery,* 1995, *59,* 1376–1381.
Katz, J., and Green, E. *Managing Quality: A Guide to System-wide Performance Management in Health Care.* St. Louis, Mo.: Mosby Year Book, 1997.

Nelson, E., Splaine, M., Batalden, P., and Plume, S. "Building Measurement and Data Collection into Medical Practice." *Annals of Internal Medicine*, 1998, *128*, 460–466.

O'Connor, G. T., Plume, S. K., Olmstead, E. M., Morton, J. R., Maloney, C. T., Nugent, W. C., Hernandez Jr., F., Clough, R., Leavitt, B. J., Coffin, L. H., Marrin, D. C., Wennberg, D., Birkmeyer, J. D., Charlesworth, D. C., Malenka, D. J., Quinton, H. B., and Kasper, J. F. "A Regional Intervention to Improve the Hospital Mortality Associated with Coronary Artery Bypass Graft Surgery: The Northern New England Cardiovascular Disease Study Group." *Journal of the American Medical Association*, 1996, *275*, 841–846.

Chapter Twelve

Implementation Strategies for Larger Groups

Megan Morgan

The capacity to measure health and to improve care is most effective at the organizational level. An organization can be any grouping of physicians with a common link, academic or economic, that can implement a data management infrastructure to support outcomes strategies. Such organizations include medical practice groups, independent physician associations (IPAs), physician hospital organizations (PHOs), practice management companies, providers in a health maintenance organization (HMO), looser networks, and medical societies.

While individual physicians can measure and improve their practices, groups of physicians can compare among themselves and to others to identify best practices. In this era of information technology, in particular the Internet, individual physicians can be effectively linked into organizations, and organizations can be linked together to produce even greater pools of outcomes information. Yet despite incentives to collect outcomes information and profit from quality, organizations require physician leaders to champion change. For physician leaders, an understanding of organizational behavior, motivation, and planning has become part of the skill set necessary to implement outcomes strategies.

Implementing outcomes assessment at the organizational level is dependent on a multitiered approach that includes a broad organizational strategy as well as a plan for each individual project.

Strategic Planning: Organizational Issues

Implementing a broad outcomes initiative encompasses organization-wide quality improvement (OQI) efforts. It represents a different way of thinking about and performing the job of
organizational leadership (Batalden, 1997). Once the commitment
to develop an outcomes initiative has been established, the formal
design of the organization must be addressed.

OQI efforts begin with (1) a clear and simple statement of
the mission that answers the question of who and what the organization is, (2) a concise statement of vision that answers the
questions of who and what the organization seeks to become,
(3) a clear definition and understanding of what the term *quality* means in the context of the organization, and (4) an explicit
statement of the guidelines for management that make clear the
expectations of the organization for the leaders and managers
within the organization (Katz and Green, 1997; Batalden, 1997,
Goonan, 1995). Traditional quality control theories search out
problems, assign fault, and attempt to effect improvement by
forcing people to change their behavior. In contrast, outcomes
initiative is based on the principles found in Total Quality Management (TQM). Thus, the focus is on the processes, with revi-
sions to those processes being based on the systematic collection
and analysis of valid data. Problems, or deficiencies, are seen as
opportunities for improvement rather than opportunities to
affix blame.

This approach to measurement and improvement is significantly different from the environment and culture found in most
health care organizations. OQI efforts represent a paradigm shift
requiring training and education in the fundamentals of TQM as
well as a different level of awareness about the importance of continuously assessing and improving quality. Thus, finding opportunities for education and training should be interwoven throughout
all phases of planning and implementation.

Model for Strategic Planning

An outcomes initiative can be developed by following a model for
strategic planning.

Developing a Vision

All strategic planning processes begin with a vision rich verbal picture of what the organization is going to be in the future. It should be attainable, short, memorable, easy to repeat, and widely communicated (Goodstein, Nolan, and Pfeiffer, 1993). Most important, the vision should be powerful enough to inspire and sustain action by organizational members.

Creating a Mission Statement

A mission statement is a brief, clear statement of the reasons for an organization's existence: its purposes or functions, its customer base, and the methods through which it intends to fulfill its purpose. An oncology practice management group had the following mission: "Our principal goal is to provide high-quality care to oncology patients within the community in a cost-effective manner. Our intent is to continuously improve the care we provide in order to enhance our position with our patients, insurers, employers, and the community."

Assessing Organizational Performance

Once the vision is developed and a mission statement agreed on throughout the organization, an assessment of the current levels of organizational performance should take place. This requires using existing information about targeted performance indicators (such as patient satisfaction, length of stay following an intervention, infection rates, and waiting times before seeing physician).

Benchmarking

When possible, the data should be used to compare current organizational performance to other similar organizations. This process provides a benchmark of current performance as it relates to the rest of the world, as well as an internal baseline or starting point for future activities. Inevitably opportunities for improvement will emerge from the initial assessment. It is also inevitable that the results of the assessment will be met with a high level of skepticism ("our patients are sicker," "the data are flawed," and so on). Therefore, care should be taken to ensure that valid methodologies are used in data collection and analysis.

Developing Long-Term Strategies

Long-term strategies (those ranging from three to five years) are developed first. These strategies link directly to the vision statement and are kept in focus by the mission of the organization. Organizations that are developing these strategies should ask the following questions (Goonan, 1995; Al-Assaf and Schmele, 1997; Lowery, 1998):

- Is there a particular disease process or procedure for which we see significant variance in outcome?
- Do we know whether our patients are satisfied with the care they are receiving?
- Are we being faced with negotiating capitated contracts? If so, do we have the data that will allow us to have an accurate picture of our patients and the cost of their treatment?
- Are we required to obtain approval from managed care plans prior to implementing treatment? Would the collection and presentation of data circumvent that process?
- Is our practice profitable? How will looking at the process of care within our practice increase profitability?
- Are there variations in the treatment process among the physicians in our practice that lead to difficulty in the care process or variances in outcome?
- Do we have the necessary information systems in place to gather the data required over the next three to five years?

Answers to these and similar questions will help form a picture of the long-term strategies required to enable the organization to provide high-quality care, increase cost-effectiveness, and maintain or improve its competitive position.

Developing Short-Term Strategies

Short-term strategies—or projects—are developed after long-term strategies are established. These represent specific opportunities for improvement within targeted areas and require the use of specific information on the organization's performance relative to comparable organizations and customer requirements and priorities (Goonan, 1995). Consider, for example, a group of cardiothoracic surgeons who have set the goal of becoming the preferred provider for certain self-insured employers within their region. While seeking to differentiate the group from others in the area, a review of comparative data has disclosed that the group's length of stay is two days longer but the mortality rate is slightly lower than the regional average. The group's aggregate patient satisfaction is 90.1 percent using a standard instrument. In this instance, the group chooses to develop a project that will target a reduction in length of stay by 20 percent while monitoring mortality and maintaining or increasing patient satisfaction.

The following questions are typically asked in this phase of planning (Goonan, 1995; Blumenthal and Scheck, 1995; Lowery, 1998):

- Do we currently collect patient satisfaction data? If so, what are our scores? Are there areas of improvement for each provider or in general that we should address?
- What is the quality of our outcomes in the broad sense, including any aspect of service or clinical quality that directly affects patients and their judgment about the organization (for example waiting times, accuracy of patient information, and patient education efforts)?
- What are the health status and clinical outcomes for specific groups of patients or types of interventions? How do they compare with regional or national data, if available?
- How do our administrative processes (such as an audit of information systems, a review of patient medical record keeping and billing systems) support the quality and efficiency of health care delivery?

Once the broad areas of inquiry are addressed, specific projects for implementation will be selected.

Implementation Steps for Selected Projects

The planning steps and the early stage of implementation are often the critical hurdles to getting started. Other chapters have focused on implementation, analysis, and data feedback. However, the steps of planning and the early stage of implementation are often critical to getting started.

Selecting the Project Team

The project team should have the following characteristics:

- Be multidisciplinary and cross-functional
- Include clinical and nonclinical expertise
- Include leadership within the organization
- Include the representatives within the processes being studied
- Include outside consultants in data collection and management and project leadership if retained

The project team should be kept small, with between eight and twelve members. If necessary, additional disease- or procedure-specific work teams can be added for specific projects.

Developing a Mission Statement and Goals and Objectives

One of the first tasks of the project team is to develop its own mission statement with related goals and objectives. This process should be undertaken for each project. Although the project team's mission statement is separate from the organizational mission statement, it should link to and support the organizational mission and vision. Its mission statement should refer to the clinical process to be improved, define the problem, be based on existing data, and set out the objective of the project (Goonan, 1995). This process follows these usual steps (Goonan, 1995):

- Develop a quantitative description of the problem. If data are unavailable, data collection and analysis should take place prior to beginning this work.
- Identify aspects of the project that have not been well defined, and provide clarification.
- Make certain that project team members (and disease- or procedure-specific groups) include representatives from appropriate departments and clinical specialties.

- Clarify the expectations of the team members and their level of commitment, as well as identify the minimum level of involvement required from physicians.

The mission statement should be in written form and agreed to by all project team members.

Selecting the Project

The initial step prior to implementation is selection of the pilot project. It is imperative that clinical leaders be included in the group that makes the selection. In large organizations, a nomination process can be created, asking clinical staff to submit ideas for pilot projects.

The following initial criteria are useful for considering a project (Goonan, 1995):

- How chronic is the problem? The design of the pilot project should address an ongoing problem, not a particular episode. Examples are a variation in outcomes for patients undergoing a treatment intervention by different providers, a long-term trend in length of stay that is higher than comparative data, a decreased health status for patients undergoing specific interventions when compared with regional or national benchmarks, or lower patient satisfaction scores in certain domains.
- How significant will the results be? When a project is completed, significant favorable results should be evident. Quality improvement requires significant resources (both monetary and staff). The results should be worth the effort.
- Is the project manageable? Measurable results should be possible within twelve months or less. This time frame is imperative in order to keep organizational momentum and staff buy-in. Carefully designed projects with a narrow focus yield results more quickly.
- What is the project's potential impact? Areas of impact include customer satisfaction and retention, reducing the risk of poor clinical outcome, increasing efficiencies and therefore cost-effectiveness, or improving employee satisfaction. Some projects have more than one area of impact. The greater the impact is,

the more clearly links can be drawn to prove the return on investment for quality improvement.

- What is the downside to the project? Projects that are suspected to become complex, overly time-consuming, or have an uncertain outcome should be deferred until the organization has become more familiar with the processes and benefits inherent in implementing an outcomes initiative.
- Is the problem measurable? If a problem is suspected but no data exist, collect the data first. Quality improvement requires the link between measurement and improvement.

Make sure the first project is a success. Organizations new to the process should select smaller, more easily implemented projects for gaining experience. Remember that an outcomes initiative is built one project at a time. Therefore, ensuring success early on will encourage continued participation by staff, physicians, and the organization's leadership.

Implementing the Project

The way data will be collected (the implementation design) should be as simple as possible, with minimal burden to the staff. Every attempt should be made to integrate data collection into the routine clinical flow. This will require input from the staff members (physician and nonphysician) who will be involved with data collection. Their thoughts and suggestions are key in designing a protocol that will consistently yield meaningful data. Requiring staff to add complex steps in order to collect data will result in data not being collected.

Before data are collected broadly, a small test should be done to fine-tune the protocol for implementation. This will save problems when broader data collection takes place.

Carefully training the data coordinators responsible for ensuring a complete data set for each patient enrolled in the quality project is also important. These training sessions can be facilitated by the project leader, if one has been retained, or another member of the project team. Keep the protocol in draft until after the training sessions have been completed; some of the most valuable input regarding implementation and data collection has arisen from the training sessions. During the training session, encourage suggestions about what will and will not work.

Conclusion

No organization plans to fail when implementing an outcomes initiative; nevertheless, some fail to plan. Whether an organization is creating a single project or crafting the implementation of a broad outcomes initiative, there is a continuum of activities, and all must be planned for carefully, with adequate input, prior to beginning data collection. A strong commitment to planning, training, and educating will provide the foundation from which the emerging outcomes initiative can become an integral part of the organization's culture.

References

Al-Assaf, A., and Schmele, J. *The Textbook of Total Quality in Health Care.* Boca Raton, Fla.: St. Lucie Press, 1997.

Batalden, P. "Organization-wide Quality Improvement in Health Care." In A. Al-Assaf and J. Schmele (eds.), *The Textbook of Total Quality in Health Care.* Boca Raton, Fla.: St. Lucie Press, 1997.

Blumenthal, D., and Scheck, A. (eds.). *Improving Clinical Practice: Total Quality Management and the Physician.* San Francisco: Jossey-Bass, 1995.

Goodstein, L., Nolan, T., and Pfeiffer, J. W. *Applied Strategic Planning: A Comprehensive Guide.* New York: McGraw-Hill, 1993.

Goonan, K. *The Juran Prescription: Clinical Quality Management.* San Francisco: Jossey-Bass, 1995.

Katz, J., and Green, E. *Managing Quality: A Guide to System-wide Performance Management in Health Care.* St. Louis: Mosby Year Book, 1997.

Lowery, J. (ed.). *CultureShift: A Leader's Guide to Managing Change in Healthcare.* Chicago: American Hospital Association, 1998.

Chapter Thirteen

How Data Can Change Practice

Nancy Peacock Heath
Richard E. Gliklich

Outcomes management is based on the concept of providing collected and analyzed knowledge to effect change. It is one form of evidence-based medical decision making. Other forms of evidence-based medicine also reflect an outcomes-based focus. These methods include evidence-based literature reviews, guidelines and clinical pathways, predictor models, and medical decision algorithms. A central question for proponents of outcomes management is whether data or evidence can actually change physician behavior.

The literature is replete with examples of the impact of various forms of evidence-based information on physician practice behavior. Not all of the findings are positive. In 1987 the RAND Corporation undertook a study of the effect that the National Institutes of Health "consensus panels" had on clinical practice. Consensus panels were groups of experts brought together to review, discuss, and advocate certain approaches to particular diseases. Their conclusion was that there was practically no effect. (Kosecoff and others, 1987; Wortman, Vinokur, and Sechrest, 1988; Kanouse and others, 1989). Similarly, a study in Canada on the effect of guidelines for cesarean sections caused little change in cesarean section rates, although doctors were generally aware of the guidelines (Soliman and Burrows, 1993). A recent study of family physicians' attitudes toward practice guidelines showed that although 69 percent of physicians responding to a survey indicated that they held a positive attitude toward guidelines, only 44 percent reported ever using any, and only 27 percent knew where to locate a guideline on a particular topic (Wolff, Bower, Marbella, and Casanova, 1998).

In order to be successful, outcomes management systems must report data to physicians in ways that are likely to influence behavior. For example, it has been shown that large outcomes databases that provide comparative data to clinicians can influence practice positively. In a study of acute myocardial infarction, Marciniak and others (1998) demonstrated that feedback to physicians of aggregated data from peer review organizations on rates of aspirin and beta-blocker usage significantly improved the quality of care delivered compared to physicians and hospitals not receiving such data. It seems that the more specific the information is on providing support for or against a particular decision node in a clinician's decision making, the more likely it is to influence change. This argues for the value of providing the end users with their own specific data set as well as large aggregate data sets to support evidence-based decision making.

The second factor that influences the value of outcomes measurements in support of evidence-based decision making is the temporal proximity of the information to the point of care. These temporal relationships can be described as distant, near real time, and real time. An evidence-based review of the medical literature for a particular treatment would be considered distant from the point of care. Reading a journal article on a particular condition is another example of information that is typically distant from the point of care. At most, a clinician can hope to retain only a few important treatment concepts from a journal article, and these concepts are rarely presented and almost never fully remembered as applicable algorithms. Near-real-time presentation of evidence-based medicine includes such things as structured clinical pathways on the clinical floor. Unfortunately the information cited may be old or may not be generalizable to the patient for whom care is being decided. Another example is that of systems that allow physicians to review their own experience, meaning their own outcomes and those of their peers, for similar patients who have presented to them in the past. "Real time" implies that relevant data are presented to the physician at the point of care. A computerized decision algorithm based on a predictor model that uses the patient's data for simulation and is immediately available in the clinic at the point of care would be considered real time. For example, Schringer, Baraff,

Rogers, and Cretin (1997) demonstrated that clinicians who receive real-time information on recommendations for testing, treatment, and disposal of dangerous body fluids had very high compliance with guidelines; when the computer system providing these reminders was removed, compliance levels returned to baseline.

There are several factors of importance in the impact of evidence on medical decision making. First, the source of the evidence will determine its applicability to the decision-making process. Evidence from a user's own outcomes experience and patient population will be more relevant to the patient to which it is applied and more compelling to the user. Second, the closer the information is supplied temporally to the decision point in care, the more likely it is for the information to influence the decision. The ideal combination would be the use of a large, prospectively collected, condition-specific outcomes database that is used to improve real-time decision support algorithms continuously. Such a system would provide the user with the ability to choose best practices within a system for a particular patient. Simulation models, for example, in stroke (Matchar and others, 1997), have explored this concept using large databases or groups of databases to generate probabilities of different outcomes for the purpose of decision support.

A third factor of importance in using data to improve care management is relevance. Researchers have shown that providing results of patient-centered outcomes measures to the clinician in arthritis may not affect either the process or the outcome of care (Kazis, Callahan, Meenan, and Pincus, 1990). Yet providing data to clinicians in acute myocardial infarction clearly does. This disparity relates to the relevance and interpretability of the outcomes measures as perceived by the clinician. To aid in decision making, outcomes measurement reporting must be relevant and simple (Liang and Shadick, 1997). As described in Chapters Two and Four, utility scales, composite outcome indexes, and balanced outcome scores are approaches to achieving simplicity and relevance.

A fourth factor is incentive. Physicians who are rewarded for participation in evidence-based medicine or outcomes management are more likely to respond to the data. One medical malpractice company has used the incentive of lower premiums to improve care and reduce service delivery costs. Under the MMI Clinical Risk Modification Guidelines programs, participating physicians have been able to improve quality, reduce costs, and thereby decrease medical malpractice premiums in the areas of fetal monitoring, sedation monitoring, emergency department treatment of chest pain, and selection of surgical patients and site of surgery (MMI Companies, 1998).

Another factor of importance in the ability of outcomes data to influence behavior is in method of presentation. Clinical outcomes data can be used as an educational tool or as a method to judge or rate clinicians. As Brent James (1997) has pointed out, systems that "judge" identify care providers with poor outcomes and hold them accountable. Judgment systems set a minimal standard. They focus on the lower end of the performance curve. James argues that the only acceptable standard for poor outcomes, such as complications, is zero. The only appropriate aim is to aim for the ideal. In addition, judgment systems lead to defensive postures, "gaming" maneuvers, and overmanaging decisions rather than looking to systems. Leape (1994; Leape and others, 1995) has suggested that medical errors usually arise from system failures combined with human error. Therefore, systems analysis rather than blame is the appropriate route toward improvement. In contrast, systems focused on learning seek to identify specific interventions that can improve care delivery and succeed in adding these to the routine process of care. The success of outcomes data in influencing physician behavior depends as much on the cultural philosophy in which it is administered as it does on the value and timing of the data presented.

References

Berg, M. "Working with Protocols: A Sociological View." *Netherlands Journal of Medicine,* 1996, *49*(3), 119–125.

James, B. C. "Every Defect a Treasure: Learning from Adverse Events in Hospitals." *Medical Journal of Australia,* 1997, *166,* 484–487.

Kanouse, D. E., and others. *Changing Medical Practice Through Technology Assessment: An Evaluation of the National Institutes of Health Consensus Development Program.* Santa Monica, Calif.: RAND Corporation, 1989.

Kaplan, S. H., and others. "Characteristics of Physicians with Participatory Decision-Making Styles." *Annals of Internal Medicine,* 1996, *124*(5), 497–504.

Kazis, L. E., Callahan, L. F., Meenan, R. F., and Pincus, T. "Health Status Reports in the Care of Patients with Rheumatoid Arthritis." *Journal of Clinical Epidemiology,* 1990, *43,* 1243–1253.

Kosecoff, J., and others. "Effects of the National Institutes of Health Consensus Development Program on Physician Practice." *Journal of the American Medical Association,* 1987, *258*(19), 2798–2813.

Leape, L. L. "Error in Medicine." *Journal of the American Medical Association,* 1994, *272,* 1851–1857.

Leape, L. L., and others. "Systems Analysis of Adverse Drug Events." *Journal of the American Medical Association,* 1995, *274,* 35–43.

Liang, M. H., and Shadick, N. "Feasibility and Utility of Adding Disease-Specific Outcome Measures to Administrative Databases to Improve Disease Management." *Annals of Internal Medicine,* 1997, *127,* 739–742.

Lomas, J., and others. "Opinion Leaders vs. Audit and Feedback to Implement Practice Guidelines." *Journal of the American Medical Association,* 1991, *265*(17), 2202–2207.

Marciniak, T. A., and others. "Improving the Quality of Care for Medicare Patients with Acute Myocardial Infarction: Results from the Cooperative Cardiovascular Project." *Journal of the American Medical Association,* 1998, *279*(17), 1351–1357.

Matchar D. B., and others. "The Stroke Prevention Policy Model: Linking Evidence and Clinical Decision." *Annals of Internal Medicine,* 1997, *127,* 704–711.

MMI Companies. *Transforming Insights into Clinical Practice Improvements.* Deerfield, Ill.: MMI Companies, 1998.

Schringer, D. L., Baraff, L. J., Rogers, W. H., and Cretin, S. "Implementation of Clinical Guidelines Using a Computer Charting System: Effect of the Initial Care of Health Care Works Exposed to Body Fluids." *Journal of the American Medical Association,* 1997, *278*(19), 1585–1590.

Soliman, S. R., and Burrows, R. F. "Cesarean Section: Analysis of the Experience Before and After the National Consensus Conference on Aspects of Cesarean Birth." *Canadian Medical Association Journal,* 1993, *148*(8), 1315–1320.

Soumerai, S. B., and others. "Effect of Local Medical Opinion Leaders on Quality of Care for Acute Myocardial Infarction." *Journal of the American Medical Association,* 1998, *279*(17), 1358–1363.

Taylor, K. M., and others. "Physicians' Perspective on Quality of Life: An Exploratory Study of Oncologists." *Quality of Life Research,* 1996, *5*(1), 5–14.

Waddell, C., and others. "Treatment Decision-making at the End of Life: A Survey of Australian Doctors' Attitudes Towards Patients' Wishes and Euthanasia." *Medical Journal of Australia,* *165*(10), 540–544.

Wolff, M., Bower, D. J., Marbella, A. M., and Casanova, J. E. "US Family Physicians' Experience with Practice Guidelines." *Family Medicine,* 1998, *30*(2), 117–121.

Wortman, P. M., Vinokur, A., and Sechrest, L. "Do Consensus Conferences Work? A Process Evaluation of the NIH Consensus Development Program." *Journal of Health Politics and Policy Law,* 1988, *13,* 469.

Chapter Fourteen

How to Market Quality in Health Care Services

T. Forcht Dagi

This chapter addresses the question of how the marketing of quality can be used in the marketing of health care services. The question unfolds into three parts: How should the idea of quality in health care services be understood? How should the idea of the marketing of quality in health care services be taken? How can quality, or, more precisely, the proof of quality, be used to market health care services?

Before these issues are addressed, I would like to put the idea of quality into a larger context. Why does quality matter?

Quality in health care is important on two levels: in its own right, as an ideal to be pursued, and as a desirable characteristic in marketing health care services. The difference between these two levels of importance is significant. In a hypothetical health care system in which no marketing were allowed, the terms on which quality would be judged would probably differ from those that would be applied in a more market driven system. Nevertheless, the quality of health care services would still matter in ways and for reasons that will be explored later in this chapter. In a health care system in which the range and the nature of the services provided reflected market forces, these forces would influence the definition of quality, and, inevitably, become one of the criteria used to distinguish among various service providers.

Quality has always been important to the medical profession. The maintenance of professional standards has traditionally served as an ideological cornerstone in the foundation of professional medical organizations. In using the term *quality*, physicians have classically alluded to three things: expertise, technical excellence, and (albeit to a variable extent) a humanitarian component or bedside manner. To this mix, academic achievement and peer recognition are sometimes added.

Physicians have also believed that the criteria they invoke to measure quality ought to be universally valued and accepted as the predominant, if not the sole, rationale and inducement to purchase health care services. This is the point at which recent changes in health care policy have proven most disturbing to the profession.

Quality in this historical and internal sense of the term never served as the only axis along which the decision to purchase health care services was made. Nevertheless, quality seemed to count, and high levels of quality seemed to count even more. The tertiary academic center became the temple of medicine, and cost was no object.

But in recent years, price—not quality—has become the predominant factor behind the decision-making process. This change has been orchestrated by the payers in the health care sector, and by managed care organizations in particular. Managed care organizations would like their customers to think that medical service providers, as well as the services they provide, are interchangeable and indistinguishable. Economists describe interchangeable products or services as "fungible." Managed care organizations would like their subscribers to believe that physicians are fungible.

The ramifications of this assertion, while very disturbing to the medical profession, also form the basis for the claim to shareholder value that managed care organizations bring to the financial markets. If, indeed, managed care organizations could show that medical providers are indistinguishable, there would be no marginal benefit to paying more for a specific practitioner. Managed care organizations often argue that the services for which they contract, or the services they provide, are "good enough" to satisfy customer demand at the price point at which they are sold. The value curve, they would argue, or the quality-cost equation, has been optimized. This logic leads to the conclusion that both health care services and the physicians that provide them constitute commodities.

These statements represent, of course, veiled and not-so-veiled judgments about the idea of quality. As such, they are open to instruments of measurement and validation. They also provide a way to counter the process of commoditization.

Physicians can counter the process of commoditization by showing that medical services can be differentiated, and that the qualities that differentiate them are, or should be, desirable to the ultimate consumer, and worth paying for. In order to accomplish this task, physicians must (1) identify the ultimate consumers, (2) determine the criteria by which these consumers make purchasing decisions, (3) match the service offerings to consumer demand, and (4) persuade the consumer that the services provided meet or exceed their requirements.

This process through which physicians successfully differentiate the services they offer, meet consumer demand, and refer to these accomplishments in order to promote their practice defines the central elements of the marketing of professional medical services. The goal of the process is to optimize the relationship between the products or services that are offered and market demand. Nothing in this process compromises the profession so long as certain safeguards are observed. It is imperative to avoid lowering the quality of medical services just because the market knows no better. That is one of the fundamental characteristics of professionalism: internal ("professional") standards govern the quality of products or services provided irrespective of the degree of expertise or the level of sophistication of the purchaser.[1]

It is sometimes suggested that all of marketing can be expressed in an equation of the four Ps: Price = Product, position, and promotion. What the consumer will pay is a function of the nature of the product or service (including quality), where and how it is sold (position), and how it is promoted. Sometimes two additional factors are added to the equation: customer sensitivity and convenience. Three elements contribute to and more or less define the idea of quality: the nature of the product or service, how it fits the customers' wants, and how convenient it is to purchase and use. The rest of this chapter elaborates on these ideas and examines how to use these principles to define, offer, and profit from quality in the delivery of health care services.

Some Basic Marketing Concepts

Alexander Hiam and Charles W. Schewe (1992) define marketing as "the sum total of activities that keeps a company focused on its customers and, with good management and a little luck, ensure that a company's offerings are valued by its customers." Philip Kotler (1991) identifies several factors that are critical to making a business successful: "great strategy, good information systems, dedicated workers, excellent implementation," and, most important, a business dedicated to "sensing, serving, and satisfying the customers in a well-understood target market." In medical terms, this means the market-wise physician understands the market and learns whom to include in her or his set of customers, what they value (in addition to technical competence), and how to satisfy their wants and needs.

The idea of competition is another basic marketing concept. I like a dated, even quaint, dictionary definition (Webster's Collegiate Dictionary, 1946): "The effort of two or more parties, acting independently, to secure the custom of a third party by offering the most favorable terms." Competition is a struggle to vanquish an opponent in achieving a goal or securing an objective. Competitiveness, in turn, is the characteristic or state of mind required to compete successfully. Competitive advantage, a term popularized by Porter (1990) refers to resources and tactics that facilitate the securing of such objectives, generally by allowing one competitor to offer better terms, or mount a less costly and more efficient campaign, or successfully block the competitive efforts of others.

Traditional Ideas of Quality in American Medicine and Recent Changes

The United States, we are told, has the best health care in the world. Never knowing quite what this slogan was intended to say, organized medicine nonetheless proudly repeated it, and it has become one of the icons of American patriotism and a reason to oppose change in the health care system. Why, after all, would anyone want to change "the best"?

The managed care revolution of the 1990s was precipitated by three major factors: first, the belief that health care costs in the

United States were increasing disproportionately; second, the conviction that such increases were injurious to the economic well-being of the country; and third, the perception that political hay could be had from meddling in this arena. Of all the fundamental assumptions underlying the shift to managed care, the most critical from a market perspective was belief that excess industry profits could be trimmed without compromising quality.

It is important to understand what the idea of quality meant in this context. Stripped of rhetoric, the idea reduces to two elements: a standard of care and universal access. Standards of care can also be defined, and again in terms of two elements: processes, or what health care professionals were expected to do in the practice of their profession; and outcomes, or results that ought to be achievable, system wide, as a function of these processes.

Because of preexisting biases, process standards were derived from public health paradigms. They initially focused on preventative measures, such as immunizations for children entering kindergarten and mammography. Process standards were quickly adopted by managed care organizations as a proxy for quality. They were implemented through protocols, sometimes called critical pathways or clinical pathways, and "suggested" or otherwise imposed.

Outcomes-based standards were not as well formulated in the earlier stages of health care reform even though, as we shall see, they have been around far longer, and from a historical perspective, they have been far more important. Measures of quality inevitably require the satisfaction of both outcome and process-based criteria.

The health care reform movement insisted that the quality of care need not be compromised by cost-cutting initiatives. The plausibility of this position turned on an interpretation of the value equation—the relationship between quality and cost, and whether it was open to change. The Clinton White House insisted that the value equation was open to change. Its opponents argued the opposite. A generic value equation, plotted in Figure 14.1, shows graphically how quality and cost are related. In the series labeled Quality 1, a certain level of quality can be purchased at a certain price. In the series labeled Quality 2, the same level of quality becomes available at a lower price, or a higher level of quality is available at a lower price. The curve is shifted upward.

Figure 14.1. The Value Equation: Quality and Cost.

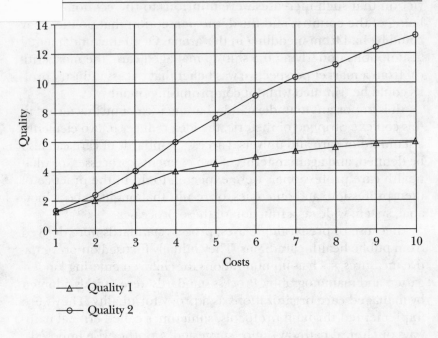

—△— Quality 1

—○— Quality 2

The ideology of health care reform assumed that the value curve could be shifted upward by certain economic incentives, legislation, and intelligent management. It also depended on the regulatory system, the standards of care as defined through tort law, and the professional ethics of physicians to maintain the quality of practice even if reimbursement deteriorated to the point that they were, in effect, losing money and subsidizing the system.

But although health care insurance is typically bought according to price, health care services are judged according to quality and convenience, two yardsticks frequently bundled inseparably. Most consumers of managed care perceive a growing gap between value promised and value received. This gap opens opportunities for physicians willing to address the disparity, but requires new ways to think about quality and health care services.

Outcome Studies and Ideas About Quality

Because of the difficulty in judging the internal processes of medical and surgical care, health care services in the past have been judged primarily by outcomes. The criteria used to approve new treatments and procedures in academic medicine have also centered on outcome studies. For this reason, it is natural to associate the development of measures of quality primarily with good outcomes. Nevertheless, the process of evaluating quality has undergone four important changes in the wake of health care reform:

- A shift in interest to broad clinical processes rather than outcomes alone.
- The transfer of focus from individual diagnostic and therapeutic decisions (the so-called one-on-one patient care model) to population-based protocols.
- The transfer of the authority to create, impose, and act on the results of outcomes assessment from the physician to the health care executive. This transfer moves the process from bedside and the laboratory to the bookkeeper and the boardroom.
- The expansion of the idea of quality in health care delivery, and therefore the measures of outcomes by which they are assessed, to include matters with which physicians have had little experience: the availability of parking, the languages spoken by the nursing staff, waiting time on the telephone, and other reflections of the experience of being a patient.

The Concept of Quality

With these changes underway, the medical profession has been compelled to reexamine its historically rooted concepts of quality. Quality is a practical rather than a theoretical construct. In the sense I use it here, it refers to a hierarchical scale of desirability. The scale may reflect specific characteristics such as the durability of a product or the responsiveness of a service, or it may integrate a whole set of characteristics into one all-inclusive scale. It is also open to, and very likely to, change over time.

There are three models of quality. The *product-driven model* looks only at the ability of a product or service to meet the specifications of its architects. The needs of the consumer are of marginal interest in this model. Many brilliant technologies fail in the marketplace because they look only at their own reflection in the mirror, and not at the consumer's wants.

The *market-driven model* looks only at the ability of a product or service to satisfy the customer. In its most principled and desirable form, this model concedes the ultimate importance of the customer in creating successful products or services. In its least attractive form, the integrity of the product or service is lost because there are no abiding standards of quality to which its designers adhere. It is this potential failing that the concept of professionalism tries to avoid.

The third model, which has no specific name, combines the best of both worlds. The product or service is engineered to meet certain internal standards of desirability, but these standards are taken as minimal only. The real measure of quality is acknowledged to reside in market acceptance and customer satisfaction, but the lack of customer sophistication is not permitted to compromise standards of technical quality or standards. This model is the one most suitable for the delivery of health care services and should be the ideal professional model.

Quality Is Not an Absolute

As these models indicate, the character of quality is not absolute; there may be several different sets of criteria that serve as standards for judgment. What matters most is to understand how criteria are chosen, what they represent, and whom they ultimately benefit.

One way to frame this concept is to think initially in terms of multiple qualities rather than a single, all-embracing notion of quality. The marketing function for health care services operates most effectively when the various qualities of a product or service are matched to both an internal standard and the proved and specific needs of the market. As a result of this matching process, the criteria of and the criteria for quality can be integrated and summed. There is no objection to marketing quality as a single, articulated concept, but one should take care not to contrive to frame quality artificially in terms of a single, oversimplified measure or series of measures. The importance of this last point cannot be overstated: the successful marketing of a quality product or service implies that it meets the standards of both the vendor and the market and that these standards are not alien to one another.

Principles of Quality

The practical embodiment of these ideas about quality can be reduced to four principles that must be satisfied if quality is to be marketed effectively:

- There is a way to determine what the market demands. (A demand describes something the market is willing to pay for; it is used in distinction to a want, which is weaker and describes only something the market desires, and a need, which is necessary for the physical well-being and survival of the customer.)
- The criteria and standards of quality accurately reflect market demands.
- It is possible to determine the extent to which these criteria have been met.
- There is a commitment to adapt the product or service to market demand.

These four principles can be developed into a series of steps that result in instruments of measurement and proxies for quality.

Instruments of Measurement and Proxies

Traditional measurements of medical quality, such as estimates of morbidity and mortality, or statistics of return to the intensive care unit after discharge, fail to satisfy market demands, even though they are important in other ways.

To the extent that a market or a market segment decides to equate a certain set of outcomes with quality, any instrument that serves to assess or quantify those outcomes becomes a proxy for quality. The proxy works only in that market segment, however. Outcome or process measurements in the abstract, in the absence of a market segment that values the outcome or process in question, do not qualify as either indexes of quality or proxies for quality. For this reason, it is imperative to determine market needs, demands, and wants before settling on a set of outcome measurements. Even with respect to medical services, outcome measurements provide a reflection of quality only insofar as the relationship between market-based criteria for desirability and the outcomes to be measured has been preestablished.

It is essential to establish whose definition of quality prevails and what that definition entails. The process of obtaining, analyzing, and responding to this intelligence can be thought of in terms of the need to relate measures to the market. The necessary steps derive from the four principles summarized earlier:

1. Study the market in which one proposes to compete.
2. Identify and characterize customers and potential customers.
3. Identify the specific and respective needs, wants, and (most critically) demands of customers and potential customers.
4. Examine how one's abilities to provide goods and services correspond to market needs, wants, and demands.
5. Select the customers and the market segment on which to focus.
6. Determine how best to serve to each chosen segment.
7. Institute standards and controls to establish how well each step has succeeded.
8. Establish methods to improve the process based on the information (feedback) obtained from these controls.

These steps require a new and far more open way of thinking about professionalism and about medical services. Because so few physicians have thought to immerse themselves in gathering intelligence about the market and responding to the information they obtain, the very fact that a practice is willing to undertake the process of examining the market and itself will distinguish it. The assembly of information is only the first step, of course. The implementational element (what one does after the intelligence is gathered and the adaptations made), the feedback loop (continuous improvement), and promotional activities will drive much of the remaining effort.

Marketing Quality

The marketing of quality is the end result of a careful process through which the parameters of quality, as delineated by market research, are determined and acted on.

Exploring and Satisfying the Market: Needs, Wants, and Demands

Suppose I were to go shopping for a watch. I probably do not "need" a watch in the strict sense of the word, because the term *need* is customarily defined in terms of goods and services essential to my physical well-being and survival. A watch definitely qualifies as a want—something that I lack and would find desirable or useful if I had it. Wants can be general ("I want a watch") or extremely specific ("I want a fully waterproof Swiss watch with a self-winding mechanical movement and a second hand, a black face, luminescent, furnished with a stainless steel strap and a safety catch").

I might have a short list of criteria describing the item I had in mind. This list can be termed a list of demands—wants for which I (or markets more generally) am prepared to pay. Ultimately demands and needs count for more than wants. To the extent I am prepared to pay for a watch, both the watch and the list of criteria dictating my choice of instrument reflect demands, broken down into greater or lesser levels of granularity.

Identifying Customers

Although issues of quality (in the strict way the term is used here) concern every consumer, the set of consumers physicians can address is usually only a small subset of a much larger pool. We cannot satisfy the entire market on all counts. Even so specific a marketing strategy as the marketing of quality requires that goods and services match the real needs, real wants, and real demands of real customers. We therefore require a way to select the customers we go after so that our efforts will not be wasted. At the very least, we ask that customers be identifiable, qualified, reachable, and willing.

Customers are identifiable when we can name them. Failing that, we ought to be able to describe them so specifically that we can learn enough about their characteristics to understand their preferences, even if we do not know their names. Sometimes several customers can be addressed simultaneously, whether they are intimately connected or not. They may constitute a well-definable market segment and evince enough common characteristics to be addressed as a group. Thus, a market segment in health care services may be distinguished by diagnosis, immediate medical problems, demographics, payers, and other characteristics relevant both to the group and the purveyor of the products or services being marketed. These characteristics may suffice to define a separate market segment.

Customers are qualified when they can afford to buy the goods and services. The word *buy* is used in the economist's sense of exchanging things of value. We must agree that what they offer to exchange has mutual value, and we must agree on the exchange factor, or price. The instrument of purchase may be prestige, access, or other privilege. It is not necessarily money.

Customers are reachable when we can determine their needs, wants, and, most important, their demands, and when we can promote our goods and services to them with a reasonable expectation that they will buy. Customers are willing at the point that they are ready to buy; at this point, their wants become demands. Businesses cannot be built on the basis of theoretical customers.

Market Segments

A convenient way to market is to think in terms of self-referencing customer groups, called *market segments.* It helps if these groups have more in common than the fact that they tend to act as a group, with similar purchasing profiles. Not all the members of a market segment may be qualified or reachable, for example, even though it is fair to assume that they all should share in willingness to purchase more or less the same degree.

The success of market segmentation is related to how well the behavior of consumers gathered into a segment can be predicted and how consistent the behavior patterns appear to be. The customers in a well-delineated market segment are very likely to respond positively to the same characteristics in a portfolio of product offerings.

Individual market segments have discrete product and service preferences. There is tremendous benefit to be gained from learning that products or services already developed can be made to appeal to new market segments with only cosmetic or nominal changes.

In marketing the quality of medical services, similarity of demands may be an indication that ostensibly different groups of customers may be treated as a customer service. The reverse is also true. One should not assume that all payers or all employers are alike because they appear at first to fit a similar profile. More than that is required to fit them into the same market segment.

Satisfying the Customer

The reason to think about market segmentation and customer profiles is in order to design products and services that match customers' ideas about quality. The question in play is simple: What matters to the customer? The more specific the answer is, the more useful it is. Thus, the idea of quality must be reduced to specifics. Is quality defined in terms of waiting time? Of documentation? Of time to appointment? Of elements of process? Of outcome? Does it reflect access to alternative forms of medical care such as chiropractic? Does it reflect a nonsurgical bias?

The only way to find out is to ask. There are groups that specialize in eliciting this sort of information through market studies. The two hardest problems are determining who has the answers and how to formulate the questions in such a way as not to bias the answers. If a practice is serious about undertaking a marketing campaign based on quality (or on anything else, for that matter), consultation with marketing professionals is probably necessary.

Defining Core Competencies

Core competencies refer both to what one is really good at and to what one ought to be really good at. The idea of the "core" in core competencies is to focus on the abilities of the enterprise as they pertain to its central, or core, business functions. But different enterprises may require enormously different skill palettes to function effectively. Thus, the term *core competencies* may include either complementary or discontinuous skill sets, ranging from the purely technical to the purely administrative and from the analytical to the tactical.

The purpose of creating a conscious inventory of core competence is to determine what goods and services one can efficiently provide, what skills might add to the real or perceived quality of the practice, and which skills add little or no value. In any kind of marketing, the analysis of core competencies is part of the optimization process of matching the product or service offering to market demand. It helps to define the areas in which the enterprise is prepared to compete.

Here is an example. An excellent otolaryngologist may have no talent as a geriatrician. If a market segment under consideration insists that both sets of expertise vest in the same individual, that market segment may not be a realistic target. But if the issue is the convenience of having access to an internist-geriatrician and an otolaryngologist in the same physical location and if collateral issues include the convenience of making an appointment to see both with one telephone call and minimal waiting time between appointments, it may be possible to satisfy these wants by the use of call center technology and satellite offices.

Another example has to do with specific professional skills. If there is an emerging market for certain surgical procedures that are not provided conveniently or at a level of quality that meets demand, a practice needs to decide whether to try to compete in the market and, if so, whether to generate competence in these procedures internally or bring in someone from the outside.

Selecting Target Customers

The ability to conceptualize a way to satisfy every customer does not make it practical to do so. As a result, customer selection is the next most critical process after market segmentation. For example, if the definition of quality set forth by a particular payer includes consultation within the same day for a majority of its patients, and if my practice is not set up to provide that type of service, I must either enlarge the range of services I provide to include same-day consultation, sever my relationship with that payer, or renegotiate the definition of quality to something with which we both can live. What will not be effective is to promise what I cannot deliver in the hope no one will notice, or to agree implicitly that I will deliver a service I have no intention of providing. In either case, I am bound to fail because I shall be graded according to criteria I cannot meet.

The key consideration is to balance both sides of another essential marketing equation: what market demands fit the products and services I can provide and what market demands I can meet by refining the product and services I can offer. The process of balancing this equation allows me to optimize a mix of products and services by customization that meets the demands of the specific market segments I have chosen to penetrate.

It is important not to become overly dependent on one set of customers. A broad customer base with different economic strengths and vulnerabilities increases the likelihood of weathering an economic downturn. Thus, the medical practice that conforms to the demands of the dominant employer in a small town in such a way that it can no longer respond nimbly to other customers is extremely vulnerable. And the practice that refuses to undertake changes required by managed care organizations in the expectation that its indemnity practice will continue unchanged runs the risk of marginalization if its gamble proves wrong. Still again, if a practice changes irrevocably to conform to the singular needs of one managed care organization alone, it runs the risk of being absorbed or being orphaned because other health care payers impose different demands.

Determining How Best to Respond to Each Segment

In balancing the marketing equation, an enterprise can choose one of three choices.

1. Change the product and service mix to conform to the market segment's demands. This option may require significant changes in the way the enterprise functions and the services it provides. If the segment chosen as a primary focus of the enterprise is too narrow, however, or if it is unlikely to grow or to survive over the long run, expensive changes undertaken by the enterprise to customize its service will not show returns. The customer mix may weaken the enterprise rather than strengthen it. It is dangerous to have a practice dependent on one market segment alone.

2. Withdraw from competition in a particular segment. If the return on the investment required to serve the segment does not meet a predetermined level, then the practice ought to examine the advisability of competing in that segment. It is important to estimate both the full measure of costs and the full measure of returns. Sometimes the promotional value of work done pro bono, for example, can be tremendous. Nevertheless, the costs must be fully understood.

3. Invest in managing expectations. Before investing in changes in the practice, invest in the time needed to approach and negotiate with the segment in question. Sometimes trade-offs can be arranged. Overall quality can be maintained while trading off performance in one area, such as waiting time, for others, such as the portfolio of services provided.

Instituting Controls

Controls are indexes of production or performance intended to reveal the extent to which a planned result has been achieved, if at all. Controls can be binary (a goal either has or has not been achieved) or continuous (monitoring partial completion). Continuous controls are much more useful in the context of a health care practice. A series of interrelated, or at least interlinked, controls is sometimes called a control system.

Control systems function only when they are heeded. Like pressure gauges on steam boilers, they are inherently dumb instruments and have no effect unless they are read and unless someone undertakes to change things in response to what they show. Control systems must also be adapted to what they are intended to disclose.

Control systems for marketing the quality of medical services must look both outward, to track changes in customer mix and in customer demands, and inward, to track how well the enterprise achieves its intended goals and how closely it matches customer demands. That control systems must be carefully designed and instituted is obvious. It may be less obvious that they too are subject to review, refinement, and change over time.

Remarkably few practices institute control systems. Thus, the existence of carefully thought through control systems is in itself a differentiating accomplishment, and something to market as an index of concerns about quality.

Benefiting from Feedback

The information derived from control systems must be reviewed on a regular basis in an effort to answer three questions:

- Are we accomplishing what we intended?
- Could we do so in a better way?
- Are the goals we have chosen correct?

The issues reduce to efficiency—achieving goals in the best way possible, that is, "doing the job right"—and effectiveness—choosing and achieving the best goals, that is, "doing the right job." Both are requisite elements of the marketing process.

Creating a Quality-Based Brand

Once a concept of quality has been generated and the instrument to track quality established, the qualities of a practice and the qualities of the services provided should be packaged in such a way as to be recognizable. This process falls under the category of branding and achieving brand recognition.

The Meaning of a Brand

A *brand* is defined as a name, a design, or some other definable symbol or characteristic that serves two purposes: identification and differentiation. Brands identify the goods or services of a particular manufacturer or vendor and differentiate them from those of competitors. If we were expert in watches, we might be able to do without a list of brands because we knew enough about the product to examine the watches on display in any particular shop and choose among them on the basis of our list of our personal wants. But if we were not expert, we would most likely be influenced by the brand name.

Brands also differentiate. In a world of undistinguished products, brands offer distinction. They serve as a way to mark products and services with the identity of the maker or vendor.

The effects of branding cut two ways. To the extent that the reputation of the manufacturer or the purveyor of goods and services exceeds the reputation of the goods and services themselves, the brand allows the reputation of the manufacturer or the purveyor to spill onto the relatively unknown goods and services. The opposite also holds true: a known, branded product will cast a halo around an unknown manufacturer or purveyor.

Examples in medicine abound. Certain institutional brands—
the Massachusetts General Hospital, Johns Hopkins, the Mayo
Clinic—anoint relatively unknown faculty members and launch
their careers. And the choice of a well-recognized figure to chair
a weak academic department strengthens the university. When the
name of a famous figure is bestowed on an instrument, technique,
or procedure—the Halsted procedure, the Kelly clamp, the
Seldinger technique—a brand is established, not fundamentally
different from the effect obtained by having a major athletic figure endorse an otherwise unknown product.

Using Brands to Differentiate

Successful branding induces beliefs about value in the mind of the
consumer and induces loyalty. It increases the likelihood of customer satisfaction. Some managed care organizations have tried
hard to brand their name, associate it with measures of quality,
and achieve name recognition. Very few practices, in contrast,
have attempted to create a brand identity, although the creation
of a brand increases name recognition and negotiating power.
Many well-known institutions, moreover—the Lahey Clinic, the
Yader Clinic, the Mayo Clinic, the Geisinger Clinic—began as a
practice, established brand recognition, and extended their brand
very skillfully.

Commodities and Commodity Markets

Competitors wishing to enter a market dominated by one or more
brands have two choices: claim that their brand is equivalent or
better, or claim that there is no need for a brand, because the
goods or services under discussion do not lend themselves to differentiation. The first claim results in brand warfare; the second
generally results in a battle over whether the goods or services in
question should be marketed as brands or as commodities.

Commodities are products or services in which brand does not
serve to drive perceptions of value or consumer choice. The purchase decision typically turns on issues of price or convenience
rather than on brand identity or other individual characteristics of
the product or service. Gasoline and light bulbs are commodities

for most North American consumers; so are the services of a notary public or a taxi driver.

Products or services are vulnerable to becoming commodities when they become indistinguishable. For example, when all available products, merchants, and services are perceived to be of uniform quality, high or low, they move toward becoming commodities. Under these conditions, the consumer has no inherent reason to prefer one over the other. The basis for the purchase decision moves from the goods or services to be purchased to the consumer. The consumer chooses which product to buy, which merchant to patronize, or which professional to consult on the basis of private and self-centered criteria. These criteria are inherently unpredictable and therefore challenging to address, unless, and even when, they reduce to simple issues, such as price or convenience. Commodity marketing addresses the consumer directly; it centers on the consumer's experience during the purchase experience rather than on the qualities of the product, the service, or the vendor. The art of commodity marketing is based on creating differentiation where none is to be found and moving the line of scrimmage from the goods and services to be purchased to the consumer per se.

Creating Value Through Differentiation

All things being equal, consumers pay more for differentiated goods and services than for undifferentiated ones. All things being equal, therefore, differentiation creates value. Whether it truly creates value or merely reflects value in the mind of the consumer is difficult to say. The only thing to be claimed with certainty is that the process of branding, when truly successful, converts an anonymous product or service into a named, known, and, by inference, respected quantity. It is probably possible to differentiate without using brands, but in the modern world, some form of branding is practically ubiquitous.

Although not all exercises in branding are equally successful and not all instances of competitive success are related to brand recognition, consumers will pay for successful brand differentiation. The question, therefore, is not so much how to brand a practice but how to bring the consumer to associate the brand with quality.

Countering Commoditization with Value

I have noted the gap between expectations of quality and perceptions of quality in managed care. If a practice were to address this gap consistently and well, if it could advertise the fact, and if it were to persuade the market that its approach to satisfying clients was unique, the practice could move toward promoting a differentiated service model. This, in turn, is something that could be branded and, once branded, marketed as a brand. The development of a brand and the marketing of a brand is another area in which consultation with marketing professionals may be of tremendous value.

Conclusion

The practice of medicine is a service industry. Service industries differ from product industries in two major respects: first, the nature of the purchase (what exactly has been "acquired") cannot be fully described until after the transaction is complete; second, the experience of the transaction has as much to do with the customer's satisfaction as any other element of the purchase. As opposed to product-based transactions, wherein the concept of quality can be separated into product quality and the quality of the purchase transaction, the transaction is always the key in the service sector. The transaction experience is the foundation on which the customer measures quality. It always matters. Sometimes, in fact, the quality of the transaction experience becomes the only differentiator, particularly in the case of commodity purchases. As medical services are characterized more and more by commodity marketing, the quality of the transaction experience is extremely likely to become an increasingly more important proxy for quality in general.

Competition and differentiation can be pursued simultaneously, and even along different axes. Efforts to succeed at one may also facilitate the other. Nevertheless, neither the concepts nor the tactics that pertain to them should be confused. Competition may evolve along the lines of product or service differentiation or in some other way. But differentiation does not necessarily result in successful competitive advantage. Differentiation must be marketed in order to be effective. Effective marketing, in turn, constitutes a serious competitive advantage.

An example may help to illustrate this point. Competition in true commodity markets usually degenerates into a price war at some point, and a price war has the potential to damage all the parties competing for market share, while granting no one party market domination. When this proves to be the case, efficient competition usually evolves in the direction of product or service differentiation on other grounds, ranging from the transaction experience, to a claim on existing relationships, to benefits to be realized at some future, to lifestyle issues.

In the service world, competition may take the form of bundling a guaranty of quality, a guaranty of customer satisfaction, or the addition of some services (which may actually cost the vendor very little) to the service mix. The pricing model may range from commodity pricing to true value pricing. Commodity pricing is ultimately limited (on the downside) by the cost to the vendor of providing the service. Value pricing is ultimately limited (on the upside) by the price the market will bear, a factor that reflects the value of the goods or services to the consumer.

Many managed care companies have begun competing on the claim of quality, a wise move for the managed care organizations and an opportunity for physicians who can deliver good outcomes and believe that the managed care organizations do not or for physicians who believe that patients, employers, managed care organizations, and other payers will reward quality with increased market share; or for physicians who aspire to value pricing.

The managed care sector has been trying to reduce health care to a commodity service. In pursuing market share, managed care organizations have appealed to price sensitivity. Because of the nature of health care, however, and the regulatory environment, they have also been required to guarantee a certain level of quality. Consumers and consumer groups are beginning to lose faith in the ability of the managed care industry to offer quality in the face of obviously conflicting concerns, including, in particular, profitability and share price. Thus, while managed care organizations have attempted to reduce medical providers to the level of a commodity for contracting purposes, medical providers who can demonstrate differentiation on the basis of meaningful measures of practice quality possess both a tremendous competitive advantage and a powerful marketing tool. The measures of quality on which claims of excellence are based must be cogent, well founded, and sound, and the processes and outcomes that meet market demands—including, and perhaps especially, the quality of the transaction experience—must be promoted effectively. Finally, it is worth remembering that all successful marketing is ultimately based on quality. The challenge in medicine today is to meet market demands with the services provided, all the while maintaining the highest standards of professional and technical performance, and refining the instruments by which to prove it.

Note
1. Marketing also includes the process of promotion and advertising, of educating the consumer about the product or service available for purchase. I will not address this aspect of the marketing function.

References
Hiam, A., and Schewe, C. D. *The Portable MBA in Marketing.* New York: Wiley, 1992.

Kotler, P. *Marketing Management. Analysis, Planning, Implementation, and Control.* (7th ed.) Upper Saddle River, N.J.: Prentice Hall, 1991.

Porter, M. E. *The Competitive Advantage of Nations.* New York: Free Press, 1990.

Webster's Collegiate Dictionary. (5th ed.) Springfield, Mass.: Merriam, 1946.

Chapter Fifteen

Profiting from Quality in a Medical Practice

Steven F. Isenberg

This chapter introduces a stepped plan to implement outcomes in a real-world medical practice, to compile the data to produce a practice prospectus that can provide a competitive advantage, and to form partnerships with other physicians that can lead to stronger revenue for the practice. In order for outcomes measurement to achieve its potential, physicians must be willing to participate, and participation is closely linked to professional and economic reward.

Step One: Implementing Outcomes in the Medical Practice

There are at least four problems that challenge data collection and measurement in physicians' offices: cost, complexity, wasted effort, and relevance. These problems must be overcome in order to establish the link between outcomes assessments and bottom-line financial improvement.

Cost

Outcomes measurements can be expensive, labor intensive, and time-consuming. In an era of increased bureaucracy and decreased reimbursement, the value of outcomes measurement must be clear to practicing physicians.

The solution is *blended outcomes*. Start with an outcomes study that will provide an immediate impact and do it in-house. I studied my hearing aid business using the nine-item Patient Rating Questionnaire (see Exhibit 15.1) and a series of business survey questions. The measurement resulted in increased sales and fewer returns by featuring the hearing aid that previous customers most appreciated. Improved net income resulted from better vendor pricing and service, particularly from those vendors that received poor ratings from my customers, because they were ready to negotiate!

Complexity

Scientific outcomes assessment requires a high level of sophistication that is not immediately available to practicing physicians and their staffs.

The solution is to *keep the assessment simple.* In my practice, we perform patient satisfaction surveys at least twice a year. Patient satisfaction is an expanded measure of health outcomes and a vital element in a quality, profitable practice. It also is very simple. The physician and most of the staff are not required to do anything extra.

I have also implemented condition-specific outcomes measurements. The recent availability of condition-specific instruments, in paper or electronic form, permits community-based medical practitioners the opportunity to participate in meaningful outcomes assessment. Implementation, however, can be difficult to accomplish if the staff cannot see the purpose. For this reason, I began with a very simple allergy outcomes measure. For a two-month period, new patients beginning allergy immunotherapy completed a brief survey of allergic symptoms. After six months, they repeated the same survey. Thirteen of the fifteen patients experienced improvement as indicated in a lower overall symptom score. Not only did the patients appreciate the attention, but it demonstrated to my staff the purpose of outcomes assessment. Following this, my staff embraced more complex and rigorous condition-specific outcomes measurement systems. Sacrificing some perfection for the sake of simplicity in the early stages will pay dividends.

Wasted Effort

There is nothing worse than designing a scientifically pure outcomes instrument for a multisite study, investing large amounts of money,

Exhibit 15.1. Hearing Service Patient Satisfaction Survey.

I. Please answer as indicated.

1. If possible, please indicate the brand and model of the hearing aid you purchased.

    Brand: *Model:*

    _____ Telex   _____ Behind-the-ear

    _____ Starkey   _____ Full in-the-ear

    _____ Microtech   _____ Half size in-the-canal

    _____ Rexton   _____ In-the-canal

    _____ Oticon   _____ Completely in the canal

    _____ Unitron

    _____ Argosy

    _____ ReSound

    _____ Other (*name*)

2. When did you get your hearing aid, and how much did you pay for it?

3. Do you feel, comparing our price, service, and product quality to other hearing aid dispensers, that you received a good value? (Circle one.)

    yes   no

4. Do you use your hearing aid? (Circle one.)

    yes   no

5. If you need a new hearing aid(s) or need service on your current aid, would you see us again? (Circle one.)

    yes   no

6. How did you hear about us? (Check one.)

    _____ Dr. Isenberg

    _____ Friend, relative, word of mouth

    _____ Hospital

    _____ Family doctor

    _____ Walking by

    _____ Referred by union/employer

    _____ Other

7. Can you buy Pro-line hearing aid batteries cheaper elsewhere? (Our price is $5.00 for a four-pack and $8.50 for an eight-pack). (Circle one.)

    yes   no   If yes, what price do you pay?

(Continued)

Exhibit 15.1. Continued

8. Hilary and Sherri at PHS have master's degrees in hearing disorders and Dr. Isenberg is a board-certified ear, nose, and throat doctor. Did this matter to you when you decided to purchase your hearing aid from us? (Circle one.)

yes   no

II. Please answer each question by placing a check under the most appropriate response.

	poor	fair	good	excellent
1. Rate the quality and performance of the hearing aid you purchased	____	____	____	____
2. How long you waited to get an appointment	____	____	____	____
3. Convenience of the location of the office	____	____	____	____
4. Getting through to the office by phone	____	____	____	____
5. Length of time waiting at the office	____	____	____	____
6. Time spent with the person you saw	____	____	____	____
7. Explanation of what was done for you	____	____	____	____
8. The technical skills (thoroughness, carefulness, competence) of the person you saw	____	____	____	____
9. The personal manner (courtesy, respect, sensitivity, friendliness) of the person you saw	____	____	____	____
10. The visit overall	____	____	____	____

Source: From Steven F. Isenberg, "Surviving and Thriving as an Independent Practitioner: The Search for Continuous Quality Improvement," in *Managed Care, Outcomes and Quality: A Practical Guide,* ed. Steven F. Isenberg (New York: Thieme Medical Publications, 1997), Fig. 14–7, p. 209. Used by permission of Thieme Medical Publications. Permission granted by Mosby, Inc., St. Louis, MO, U.S.A.

accumulating larger amounts of data, and reaching few, if any, useful conclusions. The problems and pitfalls of multisite community-based outcomes research are illustrated in Tables 15.1 and 15.2, which outline some useful solutions to the problems encountered when trying to implement multisite community-based outcomes measurement.

The solution is to *pick early wins, measure them, and celebrate them.* I am not suggesting that science should be cast aside in order to produce self-serving outcomes studies. On the other hand, the nation's college basketball elites pick their early schedules to ensure victories as they seek a NCAA bid. Ultimately they have to prove their competence later in the season. In a busy, and probably overburdened, medical practice, the physician and staff also want to feel good about what they are doing.

Start with patient satisfaction surveys. Patient perceived quality will almost always show improvement the next time you measure it (Isenberg and Stewart, 1998). I linked outcomes to my marketing and bottom line. We measured the number of patients we were seeing from a valuable employer before we sent out the practice prospectus. When we experienced the increased patient volume from that employer, with its increased job security, bonuses, and bottom-line performance, my office staff and I had discovered new incentive to participate in outcomes measurement.

Relevance

The outcomes measurement must be useful and relevant. Most physicians feel that they are practicing quality medicine. It is futile to try to convince them that they need to commit significant financial resources and time to measure outcomes scientifically simply to try to improve the quality of care that they provide.

The solution is *marketing.* Link the desirability of measuring outcomes to the profitability of a well-designed marketing program. In other words, measure outcomes to improve care, but do not forget that this is good marketing. For example, if you measure patient satisfaction and continuously attempt to improve it, market that effort. In my practice, we prepare a practice prospectus, shown in Exhibit 15.2, and send it to referring doctors, third-party payers, patients, and employers. Linking outcomes to marketing, and ultimately to the bottom line, solves the problem of relevance.

Table 15.1. Problems and Solutions
in Multisite Community-Based Outcomes Research.

Problem	Solution
Benefits of the proposed research are unclear to participants	Principal investigation explains personal and societal benefits of outcomes research, with emphasis on the current project
Office staff are unmotivated at participating physician offices	Encourage motivation through enthusiasm, positive feedback, and incentives for patient recruitment
Communication between principal investigator and data collection sites is inadequate	Physicians select a staff member to serve as site coordinator, who develops a feasible and ongoing contact schedule with principal investigator
Time is unavailable during office hours for completing forms and questionnaires	Principal investigator and site coordinators define data collection methods that interfere least with patient flow at each office
Data collection at multiple time points is too cumbersome	Limit initial project to cross-sectional studies; defer longitudinal studies until experience has been gained
Questionnaires are overly long and complex	Eliminate all questions tangential to specific hypothesis under study; limit forms to a single page or postcard
Eligible patients are not seen by a physician during the recruitment period	Define a realistic, seasonally appropriate recruitment period; add a 10–20% safety margin to sample size estimates

Source: From Steven F. Isenberg and R. Rosenfeld, "Problems and Pitfalls in Community Based Outcomes Research" in *Otolaryngology—Head and Neck Surgery,* 3rd edition, ed. Charles W. Cummings (St. Louis, MO: Mosby, 1998). Used by permission of the publisher.

Table 15.2. Characteristics of Research
by Independent Practitioners and Academic Physicians.

Characteristic	Research by Academic Physicians	Research by Independent Practitioners
Publication volume	Large	Small
Motivation	Career advancement	Self-initiative
Predominant design(s)	Analytic and experimental	Descriptive
Target population	Hospital based	Community based
Outcomes research	Suitability varies	Excellent opportunities
Funding	Difficult, but accessible	Multiple barriers; institutional review board
Support staff origin	Department and university	Private practice office
Research time	Dedicated time often unavailable	Intermixed with patient care
Statistical consultation	Via university	Limited access
Multisite studies	Difficult	Extremely difficult

Note: Differences are intended to reflect broad trends; individual variations occur.

Source: From Steven F. Isenberg and R. Rosenfeld, "Problems and Pitfalls in Community Based Outcomes Research" in *Otolaryngology—Head and Neck Surgery,* 3rd edition, ed. Charles W. Cummings (St. Louis, MO: Mosby, 1998). Used by permission of the publisher.

Exhibit 15.2. Practice Prospectus.

"Thank you for the information packet and articles regarding Project Solo. Clearly, this organization is well ahead of its time in 'mind set' and appropriate priorities."
—Gregory N. Larkin, MD

When you or someone you love becomes ill you will need to make some important decisions. At Steven F. Isenberg, MD, Inc. we can help you make this decision. Fifty percent of the symptoms that precipitate patient visits to their doctors are focused in the ear, nose, throat and allergy. Since 1979 SFI MD, Inc. has provided quality cost efficient health care in these areas.

MENU OF SERVICES

• Otology (complete care of adult and pediatric ear problems)
• Laryngology (voice disorders, hoarseness, cough, swallowing disorders, snoring treatment with office laser)
• Rhinology (nasal blockage, constant drainage, nosebleeds)
• Sinus (headache, infections)
• Allergy (itching, sneezing, rashes)
• Plastic (office-based laser skin resurfacing)
• Hearing (complete line of hearing aids and assistive listening devices)
• Cancer of the Head and Neck

Satellite location:

Steven F. Isenberg, MD, FACS
8040 Clearvista Pkwy Suite #450
Indianapolis, IN 46256-4673
317-841-2345
FAX: 317-355-1992

If your health plan or referral network doesn't list Steven F. Isenberg, MD, as a provider, shouldn't you ask why?

Free Parking
is available at
both offices.

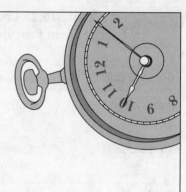

IT'S TIME...

to demonstrate quality, cost effective health care.

Steven F. Isenberg, MD, FACS

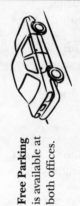

CONTINUOUS QUALITY IMPROVEMENT

STEVEN F. ISENBERG, M.D.
Outpatient Procedure Efficiency

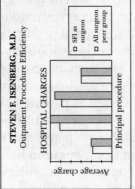

HOSPITAL CHARGES

Average charge

Principal procedure

☐ SFI as surgeon
☐ All surgeon peer group

COST EFFECTIVENESS
SFI provides quality care for less cost than other physicians providing the same treatment over a three year period. This is done by being attentive to costs, advocating for patients when they have been overcharged and providing patient education.

STEVEN F. ISENBERG, M.D.
Outpatient Procedure Efficiency

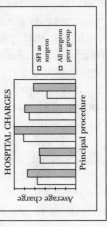

HOSPITAL CHARGES

Average charge

Principal procedure

☐ SFI as surgeon
☐ All surgeon peer group

- At SFI MD, Inc., we continuously strive for quality. We have benchmarked our customer satisfaction surveys and we consistently exceed national data.
- We perform clinical outcomes studies that allow us to continuously assess and improve the quality of our care.
- We are *independent* and we can therefore continuously search for hospitals, labs, and other facilities that provide the best quality at the best price.
- We provide thorough patient education and prevention programs such as smoking cessation, environmental control, and dietary advice.
- Steven F. Isenberg, MD, is Founder of Project Solo and Physician's Information Exchange—a physician organization that pioneered multisite community-based outcomes research.
- In 1996 the American College of Physician Executives listed Dr. Isenberg and Project Solo in the PINNACLE Awards as a "model for medical management."
- In an analysis of direct variable costs associated with ethmoidectomy (linen, equipment, labs, drugs, supplies) of ten ENT's performing surgery at an outpatient facility during January through June 1996, Dr. Isenberg was the most cost effective.

PUTTING IT ALL TOGETHER...

Experience:
- Over 17 years in the same location
- Certified by written and oral exams in Ear, Nose and Throat, Allergy, Facial Plastic and Reconstructive Surgery
- Author of numerous scientific articles
- National speaker and instructor
- Fellow of the American College of Surgeons, American Academy of Otolaryngology—Head and Neck Surgery, American Academy of Otolaryngic Allergy, American Rhinologic Society, and the American Society of Head and Neck Surgery
- Founder of Project Solo and Physicians' Information Exchange—a nationwide grassroots organization of physicians united for quality, autonomy, patient advocacy, and cost containment.

Main Office:
Steven F. Isenberg, MD, FACS
1400 No. Ritter Avenue Suite #221
Indianapolis, IN 46219-3046
317-355-1010
Fax: 317-355-1992

Measurement and improvement are intertwined. It is impossible to make improvements without measurement (Nelson, Splaine, Batalden, and Plume, 1998) and impossible to proceed with measurement in medical practices unless physicians perceive value in participating.

In community-based medical practices, outcomes assessment can be linked to income. Quality will improve as a consequence of this approach.

Step Two: Realizing a Competitive Advantage

The practice prospectus shown in Exhibit 15.2 is my way of marketing my focus on outcomes in the office. The prospectus provides not only a menu of services and experience, but data from the practice. I have sent this prospectus to major employers and referring physicians, and have displayed it in the reception room.

Patient Satisfaction and the Practice

A critical issue in securing a competitive advantage revolves around customer service. Patient (customer) satisfaction is as important to medical practice business performance as it is to quality of care. The satisfied patient is more likely to comply with physician directives and refer others to the practice. The scientific, objective assessment of what actually works (outcomes) not only improves the quality of care, but also enables the physician to repeat what does work. This results in the production of more product (new patient visits), fewer repeat visits (recalls), less erosion of patient visits to alternative medicine, and considerably less physician frustration.

Integrating patient satisfaction into medical practice management was the foundation for the national organization Project Solo (PS). PS offers a potentially valuable tool to manage the practice. As an organization of physician peers, each physician can benchmark himself or herself on a measure such as patient satisfaction (Isenberg, Davis, and Keaton, 1996; Isenberg and Rosenfeld, 1997). As satisfaction improves, patient base expands and revenues increase. The PACE (Patient Assessed Compensation for Employees) program permits medical office managers to link employee compensation to the biannual scientific measurement of patient satisfaction. This Internet-based technology permits confidential demographic benchmarking. PACE serves as an excellent practice management and quality improvement device.

Presenting customer satisfaction results at office meetings allowed me to introduce the concept of unexpected quality: the quality that customers receive even before they ask for it (Kano, Seraku, Takahashi, and Tsuji, 1984). It is this quality that separates one business from the pack. The Japanese demonstrated unexpected quality with lamp bulbs that have a mean time between failure of 1,000 hours and a videotape that records 190 minutes even though it specifies 180 minutes. Encouraging employees to seek to provide unexpected quality distances us from the rest, while improving both patient satisfaction and the bottom line.

The customer is the most important part of the production line (Deming, 1986). Focusing on customer satisfaction enables the medical office to measure an outcome and to simultaneously improve the bottom line.

Cost-Effectiveness and the Practice Prospectus

Cost-effectiveness is important in obtaining a competitive advantage. The bar graph in Figure 15.1 compares the hospital costs my patients were assessed ("Physician") to those costs assessed to the patients of my peers ("All surgeon peers"). Data such as these can be obtained from hospital information systems or from initiatives performed by local and regional medical societies. What if the physician discovers that he is an outlier (as I was in some categories)? I believe that the physician who discovers that he or she is an outlier is better off discovering this before someone else does. At least he has the opportunity to effect change. Physician participation in outcomes studies not only benchmarks quality of care, it also improves the care provided. This participation can and should be marketed, such as I have done in the practice prospectus.

Step Three: Networking with Peers

Nearly all of the revenue generated in a medical office results from the physician's production of product and service. In order to make the transition from the industrial mind-set of working harder

Figure 15.1. Physician Outpatient Procedure Efficiency.

Hospital Charges, 1992–1995

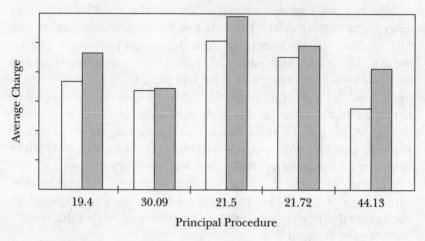

☐ Physician

▨ All surgeon peer

		Number of Cases:
Procedure	**Description**	**Physician**
19.4	Myringoplasty	75
30.09	Other excision of larynx	50
21.5	Submucous resection of nasal septum	47
21.72	Open reduction of nasal fracture	46
44.13	Other gastoscopy	31

Source: From Steven F. Isenberg, "Surviving and Thriving as an Independent Practitioner: The Search for Continuous Quality Improvement," in *Managed Care, Outcomes and Quality: A Practical Guide,* ed. Steven F. Isenberg (New York: Thieme Medical Publications, 1997), Fig. 14–11a & b, p. 214. Used by permission of Thieme Medical Publications.

to the new mind-set of working smarter, physicians must embrace the opportunities afforded by technology.

The true product of a business is the business itself. Ray Kroc of McDonald's realized that a hamburger restaurant that relied on his specific ability to cook would be a job, not a business. If medical practitioners wish to boost revenues in the future, they must become businesspeople. Outcomes assessment, or the unified efforts of physicians to record data through physician-owned databases, offers individual practitioners the best opportunity to improve revenues. The establishment of health information partnerships allows physicians to continue patient care, while subsequently recording data that have market value. These data, when compiled with scientific integrity, confidentiality, and office-friendly implementation, can benefit many who have a stake in health care. Consider this example:

External otitis (EO), also known as swimmer's ear, is a medical condition that is more efficiently treated with ear drops than with oral antibiotics. Unfortunately, for unknown reasons, ear drops are used less commonly in EO than oral antibiotics. This results in less efficacious and more expensive care and subjects patients to the potential risks of antibiotics, decreased quality of life from prolonged infection, and impaired performance status.

A pharmaceutical company has developed a medicinal ear drop preparation. It has performed the required clinical trials, and efficacy has been demonstrated. What is now required is clinical evidence that these ear drops actually benefit patients. This information is important to the company in terms of marketing and necessary in order to obtain formulary status for the ear drops. The company must demonstrate the economic value of this medication to its managed care customers. The company wishes to study the outcomes of therapy for external otitis using the ear drops versus oral antibiotics.

The company sponsors an outcomes study. Medical practitioners participate in the recruitment of patients and the administration of the study protocol. The measurements are simple but valid and reliable and are easily printed off in the office. The study forms are completed by the patients and the physician and are then transmitted by a member of the staff. The entire process takes less than a minute of the physician's time and only a few minutes from the staff. This process is very adaptable in offices using electronic medical records.

The physician realizes the following benefits from undertaking the study:

- Business. The data generated have value, and the physician is being compensated for gathering them. Physicians are now working *on* their business, not just *in* it.

- Quality. If the physician did not know that ear drops were appropriate for OE, the results of the data overall will likely demonstrate this fact to the participating physicians. The educational process that resulted as a by-product therefore improves quality.

- Marketing. The individual physician realizes that ear drops are appropriate. Future efficiencies lie in reduced visits by disgruntled patients. Marketing the physician's participation in these studies designed to improve the quality of care is an advantage.

  Patients realize benefits too:

- Reduced morbidity, improved quality of life, and improved performance status. Clearly when patients are provided with the appropriate treatment, the entire health care system is functioning to provide quality patient care.

- Value. Patients and payers are usually asked to assume the cost of inappropriate care. There is certainly increased cost if a patient purchases unnecessary oral antimicrobials or requires additional physician visits or even hospitalization due to delayed, inappropriate treatment.

Health information partnerships benefit physicians, patients, payers, and other segments of the health care industry. For widespread outcomes research to succeed, physicians must have an incentive to participate. Health information partnerships bring the innovation to outcome assessments, an outstanding *business* opportunity to physicians, and widespread benefits to health care overall.

The Final Step: Learning the Methodology

Physicians who follow the first few steps of this plan now realize that profit is possible in outcomes measurement. Following Step One, outcomes measurement is implemented into daily practice. The development of the practice prospectus in Step Two provides the opportunity to market and obtain a competitive advantage. Step Three, the formation of health information partnerships, provides the opportunity for revenue enhancement by joining networks of physicians who perform outcomes measurement.

References
Deming, W. E. *Out of the Crisis.* Cambridge, Mass.: MIT Press, 1986.
Isenberg, S. F. "Surviving and Thriving as an Independent Practitioner: The Search for Continuous Quality Improvement." In S. Isenberg (ed.), *Managed Care, Outcomes and Quality: A Practical Guide* (pp. 203–231). New York: Thieme, 1997.

Isenberg, S. F., Davis, C., and Keaton, S. "Project Solo: An Independent Practitioner Initiative for Confidential Self-Assessment of Quality." *American Journal of Medical Quality,* 1996, *11*(2), 214–221.

Isenberg, S. F., and Rosenfeld, R. "Problems and Pitfalls in Community Based Outcomes Research." *Otolaryngology Head and Neck Surgery,* 1997, *116,* 662–665.

Isenberg, S. F., and Stewart, M. "Utilizing Patient Satisfaction Surveys to Assess Quality Improvement in Community Based Medical Practices." *American Journal of Medical Quality,* 1998, *13*(4).

Kano, N., Seraku, N., Takahashi, F., and Tsuji, S. "Attractive Quality and Must Be Quality." *Quality,* 1984, *14*(2), 39–48.

Nelson, E. C., Splaine, M. E., Batalden, P. B., and Plume, S. K. "Building Measurement and Data Collection into Medical Practice." *Annals of Internal Medicine,* 1998, *128,* 460–466.

Appendix A: Types of Benefit-Cost Analyses for Health Care

Uwe E. Reinhardt and May Tsung-mei Cheng

To assess the economic merit of existing and new medical therapies, it is always necessary to put monetary values on the effect that a therapy has on the patient's health status. Three approaches to this problem are used in practice. They may seem distinct, but they are not. All of them ultimately require the valuation of health outcomes, either explicitly or implicitly (Drummond, O'Brien, Stoddart, and Torrance, 1997; Culyer and Maynard, 1997; Sloan, 1995; Tolley, Kenkel, and Fabian, 1994). Typically the common valuation yardstick is money.

Cost-Effectiveness Analysis

Someone who is interested strictly in estimating the total cost of a change in some one-dimensional health outcome speaks of cost-effectiveness analysis (CEA). The one-dimensional outcome index, for example, might be "systolic blood pressure" or a "life-year," not adjusted for health status. CEA allows the ranking of alternative therapies in terms of the cost per unit change in the one-dimensional health outcome index. But the mere ranking of therapies would be a vacuous exercise. There remains the problem whether even the top-ranking therapy is worth its cost. In other words, CEA is merely one step in what ultimately must be a full-fledged cost-benefit analysis.

Cost-Utility Analysis

The effect that a therapy has on a person's health status usually is multidimensional, and often it has both positive and negative side effects. Someone who merely wanted to rank alternative therapies in terms of relative economic merit would still have to convert the multidimensional health outcome into an equivalent one-dimensional outcome index, which requires putting subjective preference weights onto each of the multiple dimensions of the outcome condition. The ultimate goal is to be able to put money values on these health outcomes and compare them with the monetary cost of the treatments. This step is called cost-utility analysis (CUA), where the word *utility* denotes the subjective preference weights that must be used on the conversion of the multidimensional outcome into a one-dimensional index.

One widely used composite health-status index in CUA is quality adjusted life years (QALY). The idea here is to discover what number of life-years in an assumed perfect state of health is judged by the evaluator (whoever he or she may be) to be equivalent to the estimated additional number of life-years in a specified lower health status that would be expected from the application of a particular therapy (Tsevat and others, 1998). If the conversion of a multidimensional change in health status into a single measure—such as a change in QALY—is successfully achieved, one can then estimate the treatment cost per QALY that is achieved with the therapy. Such information could be used to allocate the fixed health care budget to alternative uses. The idea would be to reallocate resources from applications with a high cost per QALY toward applications with a lower cost per QALY, until eventually resources produce at the margin roughly the same output (QALY) per dollar of treatment cost—the same "bang for the buck."

In applying this cost-utility analysis in practice, one must decide whose preference function (utility function) is to be used in developing the composite health index (e.g., QALY) (Edgar, Salek, Shickle, and Cohen, 1998). Should it be perfectly healthy persons or persons already afflicted with the illness under discussion? That aspect of the approach remains controversial. In practice, the required preference weights are obtained from carefully designed surveys of representative consumers or through experimental designs applied to samples of representative consumers.

Once again, however, the mere ranking of rival therapies through CUA is only one step in the complete economic evaluation of therapies, because a decision must be made as to whether the top-ranking therapy is "worth" its cost. In other words, CUA cannot help one avoid a full-fledged cost-benefit analysis either. The argument that one merely seeks to allocate a fixed budget sensibly will not hold, because the decision must still be made as to whether the lowest-ranking therapy just accommodated by that fixed budget is "worth" its cost in the first place—whether the fixed budget is too large or too low. This involves at least a casual, implicit cost-benefit analysis.

Cost-Benefit Analysis

In a properly conducted, full-fledged cost-benefit analysis (CBA), the multidimensional effect of a therapy on health status is expressed explicitly in a one-dimensional, composite monetary measure, which can be compared with the monetary measure of treatment costs. It is really just the monetarized version of CUA.

Once again, the question arises whose valuation should be used for this purpose: that of healthy persons or of persons already afflicted with illness. Arguably the most fundamental and highly controversial question in connection with CBA, however, is whether the monetary values attached to health outcomes should be permitted to vary with the patient's income and wealth.

References

Culyer, A. J., and Maynard, A. (eds.). *Being Reasonable About the Economics of Health: Selected Essays by Alan Williams,* Cheltenham, England: Edward Elgar, 1997.

Drummond, M. F., O'Brien, B., Stoddart, G. L., and Torrance, G. W. *Methods for the Economic Evaluation of Health Care Programmes.* (2nd ed.) New York: Oxford University Press, 1997.

Edgar, A., Salek, S., Shickle, D., and Cohen, D. *The Ethical QALY.* Haslemere, England: Euromed Communications, 1998.

Sloan, F. A. (ed.). *Valuing Health Care: Costs, Benefits and Effectiveness of Pharmaceutical and Other Medical Technologies.* New York: Cambridge University Press, 1995.

Tolley, G., Kenkel, D. S., and Fabian, R. (eds.). *Valuing Health for Policy.* Chicago: University of Chicago Press, 1994.

Tsevat, J., and others. "Health Values of Hospitalized Patients 80 Years or Older." *Journal of the American Medical Association,* Feb. 4, 1998, pp. 371–375.

Appendix B: Developing and Interpreting Measures

Richard E. Gliklich

Measurement Development

The first step in selecting items for measurement is to establish what concepts are to be measured. For health status and patient satisfaction, these concepts are generally termed *domains*. A domain is a discrete health concept—for example, bodily pain. Although bodily pain may have an impact on one's ability to go to work, pain can be assessed independent of other issues for a majority of patients. In selecting domains for health assessment, it is necessary to identify a representative sample of domains to determine which ones are important for a given condition. This generally requires interviewing focus groups of patients and expert panels to arrive at an understanding of the health concepts to measure.

The first test of any proposed item is termed *face validity*. This means that the item must relate to the health domain on face value. For example, asking patients whether they can swallow eggs for breakfast is unlikely to be suitable for assessing bodily pain. Another factor in item selection is *homogeneity*. Items should "tap different aspects of the same attribute" (Streiner and Norman, 1989). Items should also be moderately correlated with each other and with the total scale score.

The number of questions or items is related to the discriminatory power of the measure. For questionnaires designed to screen patients for diagnostic purposes, more items will be needed than for evaluative instruments, where the intent is to follow patients with a known diagnosis longitudinally.

Another factor of importance in item selection is choosing an appropriate response option. A visual analogue scale (VAS) is a continuous line on which patients select a point between the extremes of the item response range (such as "no pain" to "unbearable pain"). The point is marked on the line and measured with a ruler. As a continuous measure, VAS may give an illusion of precision that may not in fact be present.

An adjectival scale provides discrete response options along the same theoretic item response range. Response options may be endorsement ("President Lincoln freed the slaves: very true, mostly true, don't know, mostly false, very false"), frequency ("How often are you bothered by your in-laws: all of the time, most of the time, some of the time, rarely, never"), duration ("In the past 4 weeks, how many weeks have you watched sit-coms: 0 weeks, 1 week, 2 weeks, 3 weeks, 4 weeks"), intensity ("Describe your pain: very severe, severe, moderate, mild, none"), or comparison ("Compared to one year ago, how would you describe your golf game: much improved, somewhat improved, no change, somewhat worse, much worse").

Adjectival scales provide the advantage of being easier to score for large numbers of respondents. When using adjectival scales, it is necessary to select an appropriate number of response options. Significant evaluation has determined that five to seven response options is the ideal number. Above seven options, reliability does not increase substantially, and below five options, reliability is generally unacceptable.

Scoring

Adjectival scales may be scored using standard algorithms, based on simple algebraic summation or using weighting coefficients derived from factor or regression analyses. Adjectival scales may give the appearance of intervals but are ordinal in nature. This means that although the responses are ordered by magnitude, the actual values of the assigned numbers have no intrinsic meaning. With aggregated data, one can begin to develop more accurate scale weights.

Reliability

Reliability or *consistency* refers to error in measurement or the extent to which a score is free of random error. In other words, it is the proportion of observed variation that reflects actual variation. As defined by Cronbach (1947), reliability has two definitions: (1) the degree to which test scores indicate unchanging individual differences in any trait (termed *stability* and determined by repeat testing, that is, test-retest) and (2) the degree to which the test score indicates the status of the individual at the present instant in the general and group factors defined by the test. This is the coefficient of equivalence and is determined by a weighted average statistic termed *Cronbach's alpha* or *internal consistency*. Internal consistency can be thought of as a means to overcome the risk that memory will bias the second administration of a test by giving an equivalent second administration at the same time. Essentially two versions of the same instrument are being compared against one another at the same time.

Reliability coefficients are interpreted by the statistic reported, the means of deriving the statistic, and the intended use of the instrument. A reliability coefficient of 0.75 calculated from an analysis of variance method is interpreted to mean that 25 percent of the observed variance is due to error in measurement. Although some recommended values for acceptability have been offered, there is not true consensus on appropriate levels of reliability. For individual analysis, higher levels of reliability are required than for populations. Typical values for measures used in individual testing are at least 0.8 to 0.9, and for populations, 0.7 is a common threshold. Intraclass correlations may give slightly lower values than Pearson coefficients. Cronbach alpha coefficients tend to be slightly higher than those derived from other methods.

Validity

Just because an instrument is reliable does not mean that it is measuring what it is intended to measure. *Validity* addresses the issue of what is being measured. Is the instrument measuring what we think that it is measuring? Validity is assessed in a number of dimensions that go by terms such as *content, criterion,* and *construct.* In general, validity is assessed by comparison to known measures and to known events. Ideally, measures are compared against a gold standard.

Content Validity

Content validity refers to how well the aims of the measure are met by the sampling of questions. Are all items relevant to the concept?

Is it a sensible measure for the task? Is it valid on face value by experts who review its content?

Criterion Validity

Criterion validity is the correlation of the measurement against a gold standard. For example, a new, brief measure may be compared against an existing standard measure. In this simplest case, there is already an accepted way to measure the health concept. Criterion validity is less direct in the absence of a true gold standard.

Criterion validity may be divided into concurrent and predictive validity. An example of testing *concurrent validity* would be to correlate visual field testing with a new vision specific questionnaire for patients with glaucoma. *Predictive validity* refers to the ability of the measure to prospectively predict an outcome.

Construct Validity

Construct validity is tested by creating hypotheses on what correlations should be expected by comparisons to other instruments. Convergent validity predicts that a measurement will correlate with another measurement addressing the same or a similar concept. Divergent validity is confirmed when a measurement is unrelated to a measurement addressing a different concept. For example, voice quality might be expected to correlate with social functioning on the SF–36 (Medical Outcomes Study Short Form 36-Item Health Survey) but be unrelated to bodily pain.

Responsiveness

Responsiveness or longitudinal sensitivity to clinical change can be thought of as a "signal-to-noise" ratio. Signal is the change with intervention in the measure under study, and noise is the variability of the measure, which is indicated by its standard deviation. A high responsiveness indicates that the measure has the ability to detect clinically significant change following intervention.

Responsiveness is determined by two related indexes: the standardized response mean and the effect size. The *standardized response mean* is the ratio of the change in score over the standard deviation of the change. The *effect size* is the ratio of the change in score over the standard deviation of the initial score. Both statistics compare change to reliability (they can be thought of as signal to noise). For an evaluative instrument or one designed to identify longitudinal change following intervention, responsiveness is a critical characteristic. Insensitive measures may produce inconclusive results. Responsiveness or precision is also extremely important for outcome improvement or management systems. The more sensitive a measure is, the greater its discriminating power is in discerning effective from ineffective processes for their impact on outcome.

Responsiveness, reported as a standardized response mean (SRM) or effect size (ES), can be compared across measures. In general, an SRM less than 0.2 would indicate a poorly sensitive measure, and an SRM greater than 0.8 would be associated with a highly sensitive measure (Cohen, 1977). Low responsiveness will affect both the utility of the study for evaluative purposes and the sample size. In addition, these performance characteristics should be reassessed during the actual project or routinely as part of outcomes management. Reliability and responsiveness may vary to some degree from population to population. Understanding changes in reliability, drift, or patient adaptation to repeat measures is necessary for outcomes management systems and is possible only by building in these statistical analyses as part of the ongoing reporting process.

Interpretability, Comprehensiveness, and Burden

Interpretability, comprehensiveness, and burden are other important criteria in choosing outcomes measures. *Interpretability* is the anchoring of a measurement to clinical phenomenon. What is a clinically significant change in a particular measure? What does a change in score mean for a patient?

Comprehensiveness is the degree to which a health measure or measurement system encompasses all of the relevant health domains associated with the condition under study. Determining relevant domains is not trivial and requires focus groups, expert panels, and field testing. Measures should identify the health concepts within them so that significant overlap between combined measures can be avoided. This is particularly true for measurement systems that include multiple measures to assess both general and condition-specific health domains. The reason for parsimony is straightforward. Patients may reject exhaustive measures as too long or bothersome.

Burden is the attribute of health measures that competes with comprehensiveness. There are two types of burden: *administrative,* which reflects the time and cost associated with giving a particular measure to a patient, and *respondent,* which is the time and effort required of a patient to complete a series of measures. Although patients in study situations will tolerate up to thirty or forty minutes of questions, our experience suggests that unpaid patients in monitoring situations may resist further evaluations after eight to ten minutes of questioning. Therefore, burden is related to successful follow-up as well as to cost. To limit burden without sacrificing the necessary comprehensiveness of a study, it is important to identify the important health domains to be studied and to use brief but reliable measures whenever possible.

Newer Alternatives in Quality of Life Measurement

An alternative to briefer measures rests in a methodology that uses computerized adaptive testing and item response theory (McHorney, 1997). This approach potentially improves precision because floor and ceiling effects are diminished. In the standard health measurement paradigm, item selection focuses on the middle of the continuum. Therefore, there are fewer items to distinguish between healthier patients at the top and bottom ends of the spectrum. These healthier patients tend to receive perfect scores. In contrast, a computer algorithm in this paradigm generates items from a pool that represents the full ruler for the condition under study. Rather than present all of the items, the algorithm is based on rules that lead from one question to another depending on the responses. In this way, for a majority of patients, the total number of items completed can be minimized and still provide adequate confidence intervals around the measurement. As a result, different forms of a test connect to each other on the same ruler. Precision can be determined by the user. Item response selects from a bank of items, which allows for connectivity to be developed between different measures to produce a common scale. Combining item response theory and computerized adaptive testing is a promising approach for health status measurement. However, it is limited to data collection modalities that can be presented to patients with the aid of a computer.

References

Cohen, J. *Statistical Power Analyses for the Behavioral Sciences.* New York: Academic Press, 1977.

Cronbach, L. J. "Test 'Reliability': Its Meaning and Determination." *Psychometrika,* 1947, *12,* 1–16.

McHorney, C. A. "Generic Health Measurement: Past Accomplishments and a Measurement Paradigm for the 21st Century." *Annals of Internal Medicine,* 1997, *127,* 743–750.

Streiner, D. L., and Norman, G. R. *Health Measurements Scales: A Practical Guide to Their Development and Use.* Oxford: Oxford University Press, 1989.

Index